CANCER AND EMF RADIATION

HOW TO PROTECT YOURSELF FROM THE
SILENT CARCINOGEN OF
ELECTROPOLLUTION

BRANDON LAGRECA

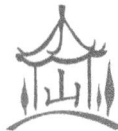

Cancer and EMF Radiation: How to Protect Yourself From the Silent Carcinogen of Electropollution

Copyright © 2019 Brandon LaGreca
E-book ISBN: 978-1-7329996-0-2
Print ISBN: 978-1-7329996-1-9

Cover design: Amanda Struz
Author photograph: Andrew Seiden

CONTENTS

INTRODUCTION

Imagine a poison that cannot be seen, touched, or heard. Yet the toxicity pervades your every day and night—while you work, while you sleep—steadily depressing immune function and damaging cells to slowly and predictably promote cancer growth.

This is the world we live in. Electromagnetic field (EMF) radiation bombards our nervous systems in ever-increasing ways and with ever-increasing potency. It is also a world that boldly embraces technology with little understanding of the long-term consequences to our health and the integrity of the natural environment.

The evidence compiled here suggests that there are many consequences, the most concerning being an increased risk of cancer development.

Yet there are concrete strategies to protect yourself and your family once you acknowledge the problem and understand the science of how EMFs derange normal human physiology. Half of this book is dedicated to those solutions.

Proceeding with an open mind, we set the stage to understand our current technological blind spots by examining an analogous public health crisis from the past. This time around, if history fails to be our guide, we may be condemned to repeat it in an even more catastrophic way.

Looking to the Past to Predict the Future

Smoking a cigarette produces a physiological change in the smoker. Nicotine enters the central nervous system and exerts its effect on mood and cognition. Smoking one cigarette generally does not produce an obvious harmful effect, but over the course of decades, the carcinogenic byproducts of combustion accumulate in the lungs and cancer development becomes increasingly likely.

The early science of cigarette smoking looked to understand these acute effects to determine whether they might predict a long-term health risk, but chronic exposure to a suspected carcinogenic substance is difficult to study, especially given myriad other environmental and lifestyle factors that contribute to cancer pathogenesis.

Decades of epidemiological research later, we can safely say that cigarette smoking can cause lung cancer and often does. Still, there are some who smoke a pack a day for 40 years and never develop lung cancer. They may die of a heart attack or suffer capillary damage concomitant with diabetes, but they don't die of lung cancer.

Looking only at these exceptions, one could possibly make the case that cigarette smoke does not cause cancer. After all, we don't have studies giving one elementary school class one pack a day to smoke for 20 years to compare with a control group of students who do not smoke. We can't govern all the other lifestyle variables that contribute to a cancer diagnosis and thus can't technically conclude that smoking absolutely causes lung cancer 100% of the time.

We can see the folly of this logic, realizing that even if cigarette smoke does not always result in lung cancer formation, the effect of smoking is so potent as to be an obvious and significant risk factor. Decades later, we know that to be exactly the case and black box warning labels now appear on every tobacco product sold in the United States.

Hindsight affords us this perspective, but we weren't always as enlightened with our relationship to tobacco products. Magazine ads once promoted the brand of cigarettes preferred by 4 out of 5 doctors.

Now we see ads for 4G networks, nationwide coverage, and smart appliances connected together as the "internet of things"—immersing all of us in the secondhand smoke of EMFs. There are few public spaces that do not broadcast Wi-Fi, and 5G cellphone transmitters are being rolled out to pepper every few blocks of major metropolitan areas.

The majority of states have banned cigarette smoking in public spaces because we are on the other side of the curve of research and public opinion. The wireless revolution is on the upswing, making us all lab rats in a long-term study of electropollution that has not culminated into a mature scientific consensus.

What follows is an objective look at the initial science suggesting a causal link between EMF exposure and cancer risk, likely mechanisms of action, and strategies to safeguard your health in a world increasingly blanketed by a poison that cannot be sensed.

1

NATIVE AND NON-NATIVE EMFS

Movement of planet Earth's molten iron core generates a weak static geomagnetic field that varies in strength over millennia but currently ranges from 0.25 to 0.65 gauss. This is the native field in which all life has evolved. The field also comes in handy when using a compass to point the way.

Understanding our place in nature's electromagnetic field environment took an interesting turn with the discovery of the Schumann resonances. In 1952, scientist Winfried Schumann discovered that the Earth itself has a native frequency of 7.8 hertz (cycles per second), and higher harmonics thereof, that are thought to be generated by lightning strikes in the airspace between Earth's surface and the ionosphere. Lightning is always occurring somewhere on the planet, and the collective effect is the pulse of Mother Earth.

Curiously enough, when the human brain is in a relaxed and meditative state, it operates around this same frequency (known as an alpha wave pattern), as measured with an electroencephalogram. This may not be a coincidence. Traditional

Chinese medicine is one of many ancient wisdom traditions that posits humans as energetically connected to the planet. It is as if our nervous system is entrained to the heartbeat of Mother Earth.

Living things also emit an electromagnetic field. The human biofield was first measured in 1936 by Yale scientist and researcher Harold Saxton Burr when he and his colleagues used a voltmeter to measure the electrical potential of the human body. His work went on to define the field of bioelectronics, eventually leading to the development of the pacemaker.

In addition to the frequency and harmonics of the Schumann resonances and the biofield of the human body, we live in an invisible sea of EMFs, both artificial and natural. Life could not exist on planet Earth without the geomagnetic field that envelopes our atmosphere like a cell membrane, shielding us from solar wind coursing off the sun.

Humans have evolved alongside other natural sources of radiation, including limited contact with radioactive elements found in natural deposits scattered across the planet. The atomic age created a demand for and mining of these radioactive elements, such as uranium, bringing these harmful compounds in close proximity to large segments of the population.

Moving into the computer age, a multitude of technologies have been developed that blanket the Earth with novel and non-native EMF frequencies of varying intensities, ranging from high-powered satellites to cordless phones and Wi-Fi routers broadcasting in our homes. With so much money to be made, these technologies were integrated into society without rigorous scientific scrutiny. Only recently have long-term studies been conducted on the health consequences of EMFs.

The Nature of Electromagnetic Fields

Electromagnetic fields are invisible, inaudible waves categorized by their oscillation over a period of time (frequency) and the intensity with which that wave is emitted (power). To give a household example, a lightbulb carries a frequency of 50-60 hertz (Hz). The electrical potential of this frequency as it moves through the electrical grid is expressed as voltage, while the power is measured in watts. A lightbulb is, therefore, a device that takes 120 volts of electrical energy and transforms it into light and heat.

Early technologies that harness electromagnetic radiation include radio and radar. These are long waves of low frequency that can travel for miles. Newer technologies include smaller-wave, higher-frequency microwave devices such as mobile phones, wireless networks, and microwave ovens. These devices vary in power depending on the need, from higher-powered cellphone towers transmitting data over many miles to a handheld Wi-Fi device that transmits within a few hundred feet.

The complete range of frequencies, encompassing both natural and artificial, is known as the electromagnetic spectrum. Within this spectrum, EMFs can be divided into two broad categories, ionizing and nonionizing. Ionizing waves cause unequivocal damage to human biology. This includes X-ray and gamma-ray radiation.

Medical science has learned to leverage small doses of these waves for diagnostic and treatment purposes, but excessive exposure can irradiate tissue, damage the DNA in the nucleus of cells, and lead to malignant cell mutation. Catastrophic examples of this were observed after fallout from the atomic bombing of Japan as well as the nuclear disasters at Chernobyl and Fukushima.

It is clear that we must avoid contact with ionizing radiation except for specific and controlled instances. The question then is, should we limit our exposure to technology that emits nonionizing radiation? Furthermore, if we can't limit exposure to EMFs from electrical devices such as mobile phones, cordless phones, and Wi-Fi networks, can we protect ourselves from negative health effects?

Although they can be precisely measured, there is not a mature consensus to what degree nonionizing EMFs are harmful. Further complicating the problem, differences in sensitivity between individuals is unacknowledged. One person may be able to operate a laptop while talking on a mobile phone while sitting under an array of fluorescent lights and not, seemingly, register any ill effects.

On the other hand, there are those who are sensitive to EMFs and may, for example, develop a headache after a long conversation on a mobile phone. There are still others who are hypersensitive to EMFs and feel a buzzing sensation travel through the arms when holding an electrical device.

What does it mean to be hypersensitive to EMFs, and how can those of us who are not interpret that experience? Having worked with this population, I can verify that their experience is real. As a clinician, I would describe these individuals as having delicate nervous systems. Tingling in the limbs, migraines, heart palpations—these symptoms are associated with aberrations in nervous system function, and they occur much more commonly in these hypersensitive individuals, analogous to a patient with a sensitive gut experiencing symptoms of irritable bowel syndrome from the slightest dietary irritation.

For those who can reliably report symptoms of electromagnetic hypersensitivity, this is a very real issue that is being explored in the research literature as a novel neurological syndrome.[1]

We are left wondering if these individuals are the canaries in the coal mine. Though they may be experiencing effects from a low dose of electromagnetic radiation, might we also, unknowingly, be suffering health consequences? Do these effects accumulate over time?

We begin our examination of the health consequences of exposure to non-native forms of EMFs with microwave radiation, a band of frequencies ranging from 300 megahertz (MHz) to 300 gigahertz (GHz) that transmits the wireless world.

2

MICROWAVE RADIATION

Unlike the lower-frequency 60 Hz alternating current (AC) electromagnetic field that powers our homes, microwave radiation is a higher-frequency wave within the larger radio frequency (RF) band of the electromagnetic spectrum. We interact with microwave radiation daily via mobile and cordless phones, smart meters, and wireless networks.

We have been assured that these devices are safe. The position of the Federal Communications Commission (FCC) is that RF radiation from mobile devices is not linked to any known health problems.[2] The early science of radiation biology asserted that although microwaves can heat biological tissue, the low wattage and the density of the human skull negates harmful effects. The rate at which the human body absorbs RF radiation is calculated and published as a mobile phone's specific absorption rate (SAR) rating. This absorption is measured as an increase in heat, known as the "thermal effect" of EMF radiation.

There are two problems with only judging the EMF effect

of mobile phones by SAR ratings. The first is that modeling of the human head to measure SAR is based on the bone density of the adult male skull. Children are using mobile devices in ever-increasing ways. As rapidly growing individuals with smaller skulls, microwave-emitting devices may pose a more serious risk.

A reexamination of the FCC standards has revealed that the SAR for a 10-year-old is 153% higher than the adult modeling used up to this point, meaning a child would absorb twice as much radiation as an adult.[3]

In addition, research has brought to light that even mobile phones in compliance with government standards can expose blood, skin, and muscle tissue to excessive levels of RF radiation, questioning the utility of SAR ratings to account for the wide range of adverse effects from even conservative use of mobile phones.[4]

The second problem is that a SAR rating only quantifies the thermal effect from microwave-emitting devices. Choosing a mobile phone with a low SAR rating can give a false sense of security if adverse effects are associated with the nonthermal effects of EMFs, the most concerning being an increased risk for the development of cancer.

This line of reasoning may have led the telecommunication public relations mill to claim that mobile phones were known to be safe when the first concerns were raised in the early '90s.[5] Of course, the studies on the nonthermal effects of RF radiation had yet to be done.

As meaningful research into the negative health effects of EMFs was published, the research literature told a different and deeply concerning story. In 2011, the World Health Organization (WHO) issued a press release classifying "electromagnetic fields as possibly carcinogenic to humans (Group 2B), based on an increased risk for glioma, a malignant type of brain cancer, associated with wireless phone use."[6] Other Group 2B possible carcinogens include lead, chloroform, and DDT.

This WHO press release came on the heels of the 2010 Interphone International Study Group paper examining brain tumor risk in relation to mobile phone use. The authors tentatively reported the suggestion of an increased risk for development of glioma on the same side of the brain as the phone was used for heavy mobile phone users and called for more research to tease apart confounding variables. The authors also expressed concern that few subjects in the study had reported mobile phone use for longer than 12 years.[7]

Evidence of an increased cancer risk from long-term mobile phone use (more than 10 years) is apparent in a number of independent reviews of epidemiological studies as well as meta-analysis of peer-reviewed published research, suggesting a clear link between prolonged mobile phone use and an increased risk of ipsilateral intracranial glioma, acoustic neuroma, and salivary gland tumors.[8, 9, 10, 11]

Some studies do not show a clear cancer association, but those studies rely on data from mobile phone use of 10 or less years.[12]

Limiting research to a shorter period of time when an increased cancer risk may not be measurable explains, in part, the discrepancy between industry studies on mobile phone use and nonindustry studies that more often publish a negative outcome.

Bioengineering researcher and University of Washington professor Dr. Henry Lai received a lot of media attention when he reported that 72% of industry studies did not find an effect from mobile phone use in contrast to the 33% of nonindustry studies that did not find an effect.[13, 14] These estimates, being an inverse of one another, suggest an industry bias that distorts the true research picture.

Since this controversial report, Lai's findings have been replicated in an analysis published in *Environmental Health Perspectives* that concluded in no uncertain terms that "the interpretation of results from studies of health effects of radiofrequency radiation should take sponsorship into account."[15]

Professor Lai is not the only one raising the red flag. The telecommunications industry has received accusations of bias and the obfuscating of research akin to scandals within the tobacco industry.

Investigative journalists at *The Nation* reported on how the wireless trade association CTIA dismissed findings of the Wireless Technology Research (WTR) project, a research effort funded by the wireless industry.

Epidemiologist George Carlo, director of the project, reported that WTR studies showed an increased risk of a rare form of brain cancer in cellphone users, correlation of tumor formation on the same side of mobile phone use, and the ability of RF radiation to cause functional genetic damage. Carlo made these statements to the board of the CTIA, urging the industry to consider the public health risk.[16]

Carlo describes the industry response to this alarming research in his book, *Cell Phones: Invisible Hazards in the Wireless Age*. A team of researchers commissioned by the WTR under Carlo were the first to document in test-tube experiments that the DNA in human lymphocytes could be damaged by mobile phone radiation. The team's 1998 findings showed conclusive evidence that chromosome damage can occur from a SAR rating as low as 1 watt per kilogram, a level below the FCC's safety guideline of 1.6 watts per kilogram. This was made possible by virtue of a new diagnostic marker for cancer development, the presence of micronuclei in living cells, indicating that cells can no longer repair broken DNA.[17]

These findings were later replicated by radiation biologists working outside the WTR, further strengthening the case that RF fields are capable of causing irreparable DNA damage at power levels far less than originally thought.[18]

The emergence of the damaging effects of mobile phone use in the scientific literature is deeply concerning considering the multiple forms of microwave radiation we are exposed to and that some of it, such as Wi-Fi, is on a consistent basis.

Digital enhanced cordless telecommunications (DECT) phones also act as microwave transmitters. The base station where the phone cradle is plugged into the wall is akin to a mini cellphone tower. This presents two distinct sources of RF radiation, from the phone itself during use and when close to the base unit that is often placed on a desk or bedside stand. Cellphone towers and smart meters also add to the RF soup, their pulsed fields constantly bombarding our nervous systems.

Many of these devices are on all the time, broadcasting even as we sleep. This is the case for DECT phones, Wi-Fi routers, cellphone towers (if we live or work close to one), and smart meters. Our bodies should be focusing on repair and recovery as we sleep, but often they do not receive a break from the stress of non-native EMF.

Plant and animal studies evaluating this constant and blanketing effect of RF radiation have shown evidence of damage in the form of increased blood-brain permeability (leakiness), as well as interference with proper DNA replication.[19, 20]

In addition to health consequences from RF transmission in the gigahertz range, there is also evidence that FM radio broadcasting towers operating in the megahertz frequency range increase rates of melanoma and breast cancer incidence via an immune-disrupting effect.[21, 22]

Proposed Mechanisms of Action

If there is an increased risk of cancer associated with microwave radiation, what is the mechanism of action? This is a difficult question to study if there are multiple mechanisms of influence from EMFs as well as other contributing environmental and lifestyle factors, such as contact with chemical carcinogens. For instance, does RF radiation cause head and neck tumors or might it play an indirect role, inhibiting the body's ability to counter the formation of malignant cells that have occurred by some other means?

A healthy immune system can clear cancerous cell clusters. One of its most powerful allies in this process is the hormone melatonin. In addition to its association with sleep and circadian rhythm, melatonin is a potent antioxidant, clearing the free radicals that underlie cell damage. Research has shown that microwave radiation is a significant suppressor of melatonin production.[23, 24]

This suggests that one mechanism behind an increased risk of malignancy from exposure to RF radiation may not be directly causal but incites cancer growth alongside other carcinogenic and mutagenic factors.

If further research supports the melatonin hypothesis, telecommunications companies will conveniently be able to claim that radiation from mobile phones does not cause cancer. This would be both scientifically and legally accurate while obscuring the fact that RF radiation inhibits the body's ability to prevent cancer.

There are of course other known contributors to melatonin suppression. Exposure to light with color in the blue spectrum (essentially any light source other than firelight) anytime after sunset suppresses melatonin production at a time when it should be rising.[25]

Household lighting is sufficient to suppress melatonin production, but electronic devices and computer screens are the worst offenders due to the brightness of light in the blue spectrum. Free downloadable software, such as f.lux, automatically changes a computer screen's contrast every evening by removing light in the blue spectrum. Some tablets and phones come with similar software as part of their display settings.

This speaks to the multi-layered nature of the problem. Not only do electronic devices emit EMF frequencies that suppress melatonin production, they also display a quality of light that adds to the effect. That said, it is more difficult to block EMFs and still be able to use a device as intended than it is to change the color contrast of a backlit screen.

Melatonin suppression may be a significant contributor, but there is another mechanism emerging from the scientific literature. This mechanism has broad and drastic consequences for human biology, elucidating a causal link between EMFs and cancer formation.

According to researcher Martin Pall, nonionizing EMF radiation incites an influx of calcium into many cell types. Voltage-gated calcium channels, present within the membrane of our cells, have sensors that detect changes in voltage from weak EMFs and open to allow calcium to flood the cell. This in turns increases nitric oxide production and superoxide reactivity within the cell that, although beneficial in appropriate amounts, in excess leads to free radical damage through the peroxynitrite pathway.[26, 27, 28, 29]

This makes free radical damage the smoking gun and increased cancer risk the bullet wound. If we know one thing about the causes of cancer, the common denominator is damage to DNA's reproducing capacity. Whether from ultraviolet light, chemical carcinogens, or EMFs, the mechanism is the same: An increase in free radicals, left unquenched, compromises DNA and more errors in cell division give rise to malignancy.

––––––

Considering the sum total of modern exposure to EMFs, it is wise and prudent to apply the precautionary principle and limit exposure to microwave radiation, especially at night when melatonin levels are highest. This recommendation is supported by epidemiological research that shows an increased cancer risk with long-term RF radiation exposure as well as the plausible mechanisms of melatonin suppression and free radical formation increasing cancer risk.

This research provides compelling evidence to limit one's exposure to EMF radiation given the long-term health risks; however, it is equally relevant to minimize exposure that may underlie acute health effects. Although less well-documented in the scientific literature, it stands to reason that anything that causes a long-term change in the body is also causing small, undetectable effects that accrue over time into chronic problems. One curious but particularly concerning example is a purported increase in the release of mercury vapor from dental amalgam (silver) fillings with exposure to Wi-Fi signals.[30, 31]

With smoking, it may take decades for lung cancer to develop, but acute issues such as cough, susceptibility to pneumonia, and loss of taste are present in smokers as early warning signs. Likewise, current evidence suggests that it may take two decades before we see an increased rate of cancer, but acute issues may be pervasive. What if these issues include anxiousness, depressive symptoms, or forgetfulness?[32] Would we associate these issues with EMF exposure, particularly since they are difficult health concerns to quantify?

Electrosensitive people may be sounding the alarm for us all. Just as there are some individuals who can't be in a smoke-filled room without getting a headache, there are those who can't be in a room with Wi-Fi without developing symptoms. Detrimental effects are likely happening to everyone present in either scenario, even if the body is not presenting acute symptoms.

We'll review actionable strategies to minimize exposure to RF radiation, but first we add to the discussion the consequences of electrification as a source of electropollution. As our demand for power has been increased by the technological trappings of modern life, so has our exposure to EMFs of low to intermediate frequency. The three main categories of electropollution in this band are AC electric, AC magnetic, and voltage transients.

3

LOW-FREQUENCY EMFS AND VOLTAGE TRANSIENTS

The dawn of electrification brought a new, non-native frequency that constantly surrounds us. Extremely low-frequency (ELF) EMFs are produced by any device operating on the 60 Hz power coming from the electrical grid. These devices, from refrigerators to laptops, all emanate an electromagnetic field that can be measured separately as an electric field or a magnetic field.

An electric field exists whenever voltage is present, even if current is not flowing, and is measured with an electric meter in volts per meter. Electric fields are dampened by a nonconductive physical structure, such as a wall, or blocked by conductive material, such as metal conduit.

A magnetic field is generated whenever electric current is flowing and is measured with a gauss meter in milligauss. Magnetic fields are not appreciably restricted by building materials.

Widespread electrification was adopted with little understanding of the long-term consequences of being immersed in

60 Hz EMFs. It has been speculated that chronic diseases of the 20th century, including cancer and heart disease, are an artifact of that exposure.[33]

———

When a number of individuals living or working in close proximity develop a similar type of cancer beyond expected averages, an environmental cause is suspected. This is known as a cancer cluster. In some cases, this can be due to a chemical exposure such as Agent Orange or the pesticide DDT. In other cases, prolonged exposure to non-native EMFs have been correlated with cancer clusters. Residential electrification producing EMFs in the 60 Hz range has been associated with clusters of childhood leukemia since the early 1960s.[34, 35]

Since then, a new kind of cancer cluster has emerged from an increasingly more common and insidious electrical phenomena. Electrical circuits overloaded with plugged-in electrical devices and AC adapters can give rise to higher-frequency harmonics above 60 Hz and into the kilohertz and low megahertz range. These harmonics travel within and around wiring in a phenomenon known as high-frequency electrical noise, one subset of which is measured as transient voltage.

The most highly publicized case of a cancer cluster linked to voltage transients occurred at a California public school where exceedingly high measurements were reported to increase a teacher's risk of cancer by 21% from just one year of employment at the school.[36]

Electropollution in the form of aberrant current is not a new problem, having existed since the beginning of electrification, but is compounded by high-frequency electrical noise.

The Discovery of Stray Voltage

Aberrant current has an interesting history. Although severe forms of stray voltage have been the cause of several deaths via electrocution, a subtle form of stray voltage was identified within the dairy industry in Wisconsin—resulting in a legal battle that went all the way to the state's Supreme Court.[37, 38]

In the early days of electrification, the wiring of buildings followed the general principle of electrical engineering: A circuit must be completed. Wherever electricity is produced, the wiring should allow for current flow from the building being supplied back to the base station. This completes the circuit.

In the early to mid-20th century, the practice of grounding wiring into the Earth itself (called single-wire Earth return) was adopted to complete the circuit using the conductivity of the ground, allowing current to spread out and naturally flow back to its place of origin. However, this practice can result in a high level of excess current that lingers or travels through a defined region.

When such a current coursed through dairy cattle pastures, a significant decrease in milk production led stumped farmers to think outside the box. They discovered that excess electrical current attracted to the cattle's metal water tank was deterring the animals from drinking. The cattle would either experience an electrical shock or generalized buzzing when trying to drink. The cows became dehydrated, leading to a decrease in milk production. Research studies examining the impact on milk production are mixed, though some mechanism involving stray voltage is generally recognized in the industry as being deleterious to herd health.[39]

Once this insidious form of stray voltage was identified, in part due to litigation within the dairy industry, concerned electrical engineers devised methods to measure and remedy aberrant current within the wiring of freestanding buildings. Faulty wiring or overcharge within the circuits has the potential to persist and reverberate through the building. The problem of stray voltage within a freestanding building is somewhat solved in modern electrification, mitigated by the incorporation of a neutral return and strict adherence to the electrical code. Stray voltage resulting from the introduction of current into the Earth from electrical distribution (also known as ground currents) will still persist due to the multi-grounded neutral system that is universally used for power distribution in the United States. Another form of aberrant current exists as transient voltage, higher-frequency harmonics of AC current in the kilohertz and low megahertz range.

Voltage Transients

Referred to colloquially as "dirty electricity," transient voltage denotes an excess electrical current without a place to go. Transient voltage is only one type of high-frequency noise that exists in electrical wiring. Of all the frequencies of electrical and magnetic fields that may be generated, the most common instrumentation available only measures conducted transient voltage traveling along the wiring, acting as a

surrogate metric of the total burden of high-frequency electropollution.

In the case of an overloaded circuit, transient voltage will
reverberate throughout the circuit and bleed into the air space.
One location where this occurs is at a dimmer switch. When
the potentiometer of a dimmer switch is dialed down, it is
restricting current that may overcharge the electrical circuit.

Electric ballasts of fluorescent bulbs also have the potential to produce transient voltage as they modulate the current
entering the bulb. As 60 Hz AC is transformed into direct
current (DC), the excess ungrounded current persists along the
circuit as a higher-frequency harmonic.

If the number and type of electrical devices plugged into
the circuits of a building generate a large amount of electrical
noise, the overcharge reverberates within the circuits, causing
the entire building to imperceptibly buzz. Transient voltage
can be precisely measured at the outlets along each circuit.
The problem is compounded when a number of electrical
devices are plugged in and pulling current along the same
circuit.

Older homes can be prone to transient voltage as the
circuits become overloaded with modern electrical devices
that may not yet have been invented when these homes were
designed. New homes tend to have fewer problems, but even
with updated wiring and circuit breakers, newer buildings can
still register voltage transients from other buildings in close
proximity. Housing density produces a transient voltage
problem as the combined electrical service in an area over-
taxes the Earth's ability to dissipate the current.

———

As we are not cattle getting buzzed every time we visit the water trough, we turn to research literature to expose the documented health risks of electropollution. The first startling realization is that, similar to microwave radiation, ELF EMFs affect calcium within the cell and depress melatonin production.[40, 41, 42]

These effects provide clues to why we have seen increased rates of childhood leukemia in connection with ELF EMFs as well as animal studies showing significant carcinogenic effects in mammary glands and heart tissue along with an increased incidence of lymphomas and leukemias.[43, 44]

Suppression of melatonin levels has been known to augment formation of several cancer types, including breast cancer, prostate cancer, and melanoma; this effect on pineal gland function has been observed with 60 Hz electric and magnetic fields.[45, 46]

Collectively, this research paints a bleak picture of electrification in general as 60 Hz electrical fields surround us in every building connected to the electrical grid, compounded by voltage transients bleeding higher harmonic fields out from the walls and into living spaces.

Those who claim negative health effects from EMFs identify sources of electropollution such as transient voltage as a cause or contributor to chronic, recalcitrant health problems. Anyone suffering from an unusual array of symptoms that improve in a different environment should have the building in question tested for transient voltage in addition to ELF electrical and magnetic fields as one element of a complete home inspection. That inspection might also include environmental testing for radon, mold, and carbon monoxide.

4

RESILIENCE

Having examined the health risks associated with exposure to non-native EMFs, we now turn our attention to simple, actionable strategies to protect you and your family. These strategies are divided into three categories: avoidance, remediation, and shielding. Of the three, avoidance is the best means to reduce risk. However, those needing or wanting to interact with technology will have to rely on a combination of remediation and shielding to safeguard their health.

Although we would all benefit from adopting a precautionary stance for the sake of prevention, individuals suffering from serious health challenges (especially cancer) may choose comprehensive limitation of exposure to the least amount possible.

Before detailing these three strategies for altering the physical environment to reduce exposure to EMFs, we should first consider how the body can benefit from building resilience. If the ability to change the external environment is limited, attending to our internal environment is the only option but one that can provide great benefit. This is contingent on the overall health of the individual and how pervasive electropollution and other environmental stressors are.

If we consider exposure to all externally present or internally generated stress as occupying a bell-shaped curve, a certain amount is normal and necessary for maintaining human health. Phytonutrient-rich plants produce chemical compounds to defend themselves from predation. While an excess of these chemicals can damage the body, small amounts challenge the body to upregulate its detoxification enzymes, protecting against cancer development.[47]

This concept, known as hormesis, asserts that the dose determines whether a substance is helpful or harmful. Too much is not good, but a lack of environmental stress also results in health consequences as the body does not receive the impulse to adapt and grow stronger.

It is a similar story with exercise. The right amount taxes the body sufficiently to grow stronger, while excess exertion without adequate recovery can lead to exhaustion, systemic inflammation, and a breakdown of muscle tissue.

It is through this lens that we should view all environmental stressors we encounter in regard to our overall health. Resilience is a sum total game. If our diet is poor and our sleep disturbed, other sources of stress, whether as overt and self-inflicted as smoking or as silent and insidious as electropollution, will compound our weakened state and may present as negative health consequences.

We may remark upon the large event that gets our attention, such as a heart attack or cancer diagnosis, but fail to see the incremental stresses that have contributed to that dramatic moment that had been years in the making.

Electropollution is one such stress, and in conjunction with other resilience-degrading behaviors and environments, it can be the last straw that breaks the camel's back, presenting itself as a significant health crisis. Thinking in this vein explains why some diseases, such as cancer, can be difficult to pin to a single cause. If we define cancer as a disease process of manifold internal and external stressors that develops over the course of years, building resilience then becomes a main preventive strategy.

In some instances, one physiological stressor may be more significant than initially thought. This was the case with smoking and lung cancer and, as epidemiological evidence suggests, microwave radiation and brain cancer.

In other instances, we have evidence that hints at an effect, but a pattern does not emerge. One individual may develop a malignancy, while others in the same environment do not. Compromised resilience and the diverse influences that dovetail with a person's unique biochemistry create the perfect storm of a cancer diagnosis while the rest of us are left blindsided.

Holistic medicine posits that restoring balance to the body and building resilience is the most sensible long-term strategy for disease states that do not appear to have a single obvious causative agent. The problem with EMFs is that few people associate acute symptoms such as fatigue, headache, and insomnia with exposure to EMFs, yet these are the same symptoms attributed to electropollution by those claiming to be electrosensitive.

The majority of the population is not receiving (or at least, not perceiving) negative feedback in the form of acute symptoms to guide avoidance of non-native EMFs. Most people must rely on the evidence presented thus far to challenge the notion of adopting technology without considering potential long-term negative health effects. With this in mind, we would all do well to apply the precautionary principle; work toward building resilience; and adopt the avoidance, remediation, and shielding strategies that follow.

————

Aside from the resilience-building wisdom of a healthy diet and lifestyle (beyond the scope of this work but visit www.westonaprice.org for a primer), a few specific strategies can be employed once the aforementioned mechanisms underlying EMF distortion of human physiology are understood.

Given the weight of evidence attributing EMF exposure to excessive intracellular calcium influx, any strategy to cycle calcium extracellularly or slow its inward movement would be of therapeutic value. Pharmaceutically, this tweak of cellular biology has long been in existence in the form of calcium channel blocker drugs. That said, good luck convincing a physician to prescribe a low dose of a calcium channel blocker drug to hedge the long-term effects of EMF exposure.

An alternative may be nature's calcium channel blocker, magnesium. Although this has not been studied in the context of electropollution, magnesium is known to have a balancing effect on calcium utilization in the body. It is reasonable to assert that a sufficient dose of oral or transdermal magnesium may have a mitigating effect on the calcium-disrupting action of EMFs. We don't yet know what form or dose is most efficacious to achieve this effect.

Considering that magnesium supplementation is exceedingly safe (with too high a dose resulting in diarrhea or loose stools as the body purges the excess), a dose of 200-400 mg of magnesium in the form of citrate, lactate, or L-threonate is generally very well-tolerated.

Depletion of magnesium in soil has led to widespread dietary deficiency of this essential mineral. This in turn may be predisposing us to the negative effects of electropollution.

For repletion, one strategy used by holistic medical practitioners is to gradually increase the dose of magnesium until a patient develops loose stools (called "titrating to bowel tolerance") and then recommend a dose just below that threshold at which presumably the patient is absorbing and utilizing the total intake of magnesium.

The other aforementioned mechanism of harm from EMF exposure is suppression of melatonin synthesis. Aware of this effect, holistic medical practitioners have relied on low-dose melatonin supplementation (usually at a dose of 1–3 mg every night) as a preventative strategy for high-risk populations. Moreover, research in oncology has identified higher doses of melatonin (20–40 mg a day) as a potential therapeutic agent for some cancer subtypes.[48]

At a low dose, supplemental melatonin is generally regarded as safe, has antioxidant benefits, and can improve sleep quality. Oral supplementation of melatonin may safeguard those in high-risk electropollution environments, but without clinical research to verify this effect, the use of supplemental melatonin remains speculative.

Finally, as an herbalist, I have to put in a vote for ginkgo. It may turn out to be a key herb to build resilience against EMF stress. Ginkgo is an ancient herb, thriving since the time of the dinosaurs, that has fascinating adaptive-like benefits on the body. Having withstood millennia of environmental pressures (including a few large trees that survived the fallout at Hiroshima[49]), biochemical research has revealed that flavonoids in ginkgo extract exhibit antioxidant and neuroprotective effects.

One study has shown that gingko extract prevented oxidative stress in the brains of rats exposed to 900 MHz of RF radiation (a frequency common to mobile phones) at a rate of one hour a day for seven straight days.[50]

Perhaps ingesting ginkgo allows us to incorporate its evolutionary-honed resilience into our own bodies? For maintenance, I typically recommend a twice-daily dose of a whole plant extract of ginkgo standardized to contain at least 10 mg of ginkgo flavonglycosides.

Building resilience is about reinforcing wellness rather than treating illness. Holistic medicine practitioners are the wisdom carriers of this paradigm, humbly teaching the laws of nature.

We peacefully remind our patients that humans cannot disobey nature for very long without consequences to our health and sanity. Sleeping poorly for a few nights and compensating with caffeine won't result in too much fallout, but burn the candle on both ends for long stretches and no amount of stimulants will prevent the ensuing crash.

So too must we exercise wisdom with our reliance on technology, placing limitations on use if it robs us of resilience and interferes with our relationships.

The recommendations detailed here are provided in acknowledgement of the fact that technological integration into society is a rolling freight train on a nonstop course into the future. Alongside other resilience-building and avoidance strategies, perhaps taking these actions will be sufficient to safeguard the majority of us from the greater thrust of negative consequences of electropollution.

5

AVOIDANCE STRATEGIES

In the sea of EMFs that we are immersed in, the sensible strategy is to stick to the shoreline. Practically speaking, this means the farther away from the source of electropollution, the lower the assumed risk. Many EMFs decrease exponentially with distance; simply moving a few feet away from the epicenter greatly reduces the strength of the signal that one is exposed to.

In some instances all that is required is a change in habit, such as setting a mobile phone to airplane mode when carried. Sometimes a little furniture rearrangement gets the job done, such as moving a desk a few feet away from a filled power strip. The most difficult EMF sources to avoid are cellphone towers and smart meters, for which placement is controlled by telecommunications and energy companies.

Mobile and Cordless Phones

With a mobile phone, the most foolproof strategy is shutting it off or placing it in airplane mode when not in use. If it must be continuously operational, place it as far away from the body as possible. This can be as simple as affixing the phone to a car's dashboard while driving or placing the phone at the far corner of a desk while working. When walking, a phone is best placed in a briefcase, backpack, or purse to provide some degree of separation.

The least desirable option to carry an operational mobile phone is in contact with the body, but in that instance, placing the phone in a back pocket is the least harmful. Front pants pockets should be avoided to safeguard the reproductive organs. It is particularly troubling to see a woman place a mobile phone in her bra, considering the increased risk of breast cancer from RF fields.[51]

Mobile phones should not be placed close to a bed. Keep them in airplane mode or, ideally, shut off while sleeping. A landline wired to a cordless DECT phone should not be placed in the bedroom. Better yet, add a plug-in timer so that cordless phones shut off when those in the home are asleep. If there is a concern about having an active phone in case of an emergency, have one or more corded phones plugged into phone jacks and ready for use at any hour. For those without a landline who must leave their mobile phone operational at night, place the phone at least 15 feet away.

When talking on a mobile phone, the best avoidance strategy is to switch to speakerphone and keep the device several inches from the head. The same rule applies with cordless DECT phones. When speakerphone is not practical for security or privacy reasons, an air tube headset that channels sound through a hollow plastic tube (similar to a stethoscope) is a good option. Wired headsets and Bluetooth earpieces sidestep the thermal effect of RF radiation but still transmit EMFs to the head and should be avoided.

Wireless and Radiofrequency Devices

Internet access is best achieved through wired network cables so that wireless networks can be avoided. There are resources available that detail how to convert devices designed to work wirelessly, such as a tablet, to access the internet through a wired connection.[52] This is especially important for someone recovering from a serious illness, such as cancer.

When designing completely wired internet access in a home or office with network cables, ensure the Wi-Fi functionality of the router and modem is disabled. These devices are often set up to transmit by default and must be individually reset to not transmit RF.

The one current exception to this are modems provided by Comcast. When the wireless is turned off via the controlling software, it will appear to not be transmitting; however, that does not completely disable RF radiation. Comcast must be contacted to remotely turn off a wireless transmission the company keeps active to supplement cellular service. In essence, the modem is acting as an access point for other Comcast customers in the vicinity, all unbeknownst to the customer.

Computers, laptops, and tablets also need to be placed in airplane mode. Even though there is no transmission for them to receive, if Wi-Fi and Bluetooth are still operational on the devices, they will continue to be operational as they constantly search for an RF signal.

If a Wi-Fi router must be used to transmit RF, place the router several feet away from any occupied space. With the idea of keeping all electronics together, many Wi-Fi routers end up plugged into power strips alongside computers and printers in an office setting. This creates an EMF hot spot adjacent to a desk that may be in use for several hours a day, exposing the individual to a number of sources of EMFs.

Sometimes the basement is the best option for a Wi-Fi router. It can be placed adjacent to a cable box or fiber-optic connection, provided the room above is not a bedroom or commonly occupied space.

Wi-Fi routers should also be powered down at night when not in use. Adding a plug-in timer between a wireless router and the outlet automatically lowers electropollution. This is the most convenient solution, safeguarding your family during the most vulnerable biological timeframe. Set a timer to shut off any broadcasting devices (such as Wi-Fi routers and cordless phones) at bedtime or, better yet, stop using all devices an hour or two before bedtime, when our nervous systems are winding down. This encourages a peaceful transition to sleep by avoiding the melatonin-suppressing stimulation from a bright screen and EMFs.

When visiting a public space with a Wi-Fi network, it is usually easy to spot where a wireless router is located and choose to sit farther away. Check the ceiling in establishments such as a library or cafe, and look for a square box with one or more green lights. In hotels, routers are often on hallway ceilings. Look around before settling in, and ask to be moved to a different room if a wireless router is right outside the door of the room.

Other Wi-Fi enabled devices include smart appliances and home entertainment centers. Anything labeled "smart" and connected together via the internet is communicating in the RF band. This includes televisions, thermostats, video game consoles, refrigerators, washers, dryers, and a litany of kitchen appliances. Pretty soon, there won't be a square inch of a modern home that isn't buzzing with microwave radiation.

Microwave ovens are not supposed to leak microwave radiation, but I have measured pristine-looking microwave ovens that pinned my RF meter several feet away. Pressure cookers and convection ovens can heat food just as fast, so there is no reason to own a microwave oven.

Another RF device common in homes of new parents is a baby monitor that, with rare exception, is constantly broadcasting when operational. This is even more worrisome considering that these monitors are usually placed close to a crib in order to detect the slightest sound. There are precious few baby monitors commercially available that only turn on and transmit when a sound is detected, shutting off after a few moments when the sound ceases. When our family was researching a voice-activated baby monitor several years ago, the Angelcare model AC420 was the only one available.

A better alternative to a baby monitor is a wired webcam that carries a video and audio feed to a computer or laptop.

Cellphone Towers

Cellphone towers cannot be moved, so the best choice is to move away from them. The rule is based on the line of sight: If the cellphone tower is visible, the proximity is too close. Tree coverage does help, but even if a tower is not visible, the most conservative estimated reasonably safe distance is at least a half mile, though a full mile is preferred. For FM, AM, and TV broadcast towers, a mile is the minimum safe distance.

If moving away from a cellphone or broadcast tower is not an option, consult with an EMF inspector trained in building remediation using shielding strategies. This must be done to precise specifications and may include window treatments, special interior wall paint, and shielding fabric draped over one's bed to create an EMF-excluding Faraday cage. These strategies are beyond the scope of this book and must be instituted by a qualified inspector with the appropriate EMF-measuring devices to ensure success.

Electric Meters

Some people are lucky enough to have an old analog meter on their property. Others have devices that transmit data from the house to the street, where a vehicle from the utility company receives usage data. These are technically not smart meters but still generate a pulsed signal of microwave radiation. These digital meters can reside in a nontransmitting state (being "awoken" when a signal is required from the utility company), though many of them are set and left in a "bubble-up" mode in which they pulse a signal every few seconds.

This will be apparent when looking at the face of the meter, because it will show this intermittent transmission on the display, usually as a set of dashes or zeros.

Smart meters are similar in design but much stronger in power as they transmit data in the microwave band over many miles. It is no surprise that an increase in health problems has become associated with the proliferation of these more powerful devices. Such symptoms include insomnia, fatigue, headaches, tinnitus, and dizziness.[53]

One could petition the utility company to replace a digital smart meter with an older analog one. This will likely be met with great opposition; however, many homeowners have prevailed. In some cases, entire communities have either had smart meters removed from their homes or halted further installation by establishing a citizen's right to opt out. Fountain, Colorado, and Port Angeles, Washington, are two such success stories.

If you are stuck with a smart meter, note where it is on the outside of the home and avoid the area inside the wall from where it operates. EMF inspectors use an RF meter to show clients the spike that occurs every few seconds in the room and how far out that signal is of significance.

The signal from a lower-powered digital meter can be detected inside the room adjacent to where the meter is externally placed, while the stronger signals from smart meters encroach farther into the interior of the building. This is not the ideal room for a bedroom or wall for a desk or couch.

The worst scenario is a bank of smart meters on the outside wall of a bedroom in a multiunit dwelling. This room would receive a potent blast of microwave radiation with the output of all the meters combined.

In addition to emitting an RF signal, an electric meter is the point where all electricity enters the home before branching out through the building. This area is, therefore, a source of elevated magnetic fields and transient voltage that can extend several feet into the adjacent room. Although the radiation could be shielded, the best strategy is to avoid this area entirely.

Household AC Electrical Devices and Appliances

AC electric fields permeate wired buildings and any electrical devices connected to them. Electrical fields cannot be completely mitigated without shielding walls, ceilings, and floors. In some cases, electric fields may be reduced by keeping as little plugged into outlets as possible. This is especially important in a bedroom.

Sources of AC magnetic fields include outdoor power lines, wiring defects, electrical code violations, improper grounding, and electrical devices and appliances. AC magnetic fields (but not electric fields) can be measured with a gauss meter.

The main avoidance strategy for 60 Hz EMFs is distance from the source; magnetic field strength decreases exponentially with distance, and fields from electrical defects decrease linearly. Begin by assessing frequently occupied areas around the home and office.

Basic gauss and electric meters will be able to show when a lamp next to a reading chair or alarm clock on a bedside stand is too close to the head. The body should be exposed to less than 2 milligauss (mG) and preferably less than 1 mG for any EMF exposure longer than a few minutes. The closer to zero the better, and that might be achievable simply by moving the EMF source a few inches away.

A good rule of thumb is: If with arms stretched out the electrical device can be reached, it is too close. Position alarm clocks some distance away, even if it means having to get up and out of bed to hit the snooze button. (Isn't that the point of an alarm clock, to get out of bed?)

Keep in mind that distance is the key. At 6 inches away, a small plug-in hair dryer registers 15 mG on low and pins my gauss meter at more than 100 mG on high. Change the distance to 12 inches, and the low setting drops down to 2 mG while the high setting only tops out at 3 mG. Almost all hair dryers are a prominent source of electropollution because they expose the head to intense radiation, even if only for a brief time. Because some of my patients who are prone to headaches or migraines have reported an increased incidence of head pain following hair dryer use, I recommend against regular use of hair dryers.

With some electrical devices, such as a laptop, there is an appreciable EMF field both when using it plugged in and when it is operating on battery power. When I placed my gauss meter on top of my laptop keyboard while typing this text, the meter would regularly spike, pinning the needle in the upper range of 100 mG regardless of whether the adapter cable was plugged in (though the field strength increased when plugged in). This EMF field is generated by the circuitry of the computer as it processes. Working on an external USB-wired keyboard will significantly reduce electropollution that comes in contact with the hands.

In other cases, operating a device on battery power exposes the user to weaker EMFs. When turned on, my electric razor registers 5 mG on battery and doubles to 10 mG when plugged in.

Consider purchasing a professional gauss meter to locate EMF hot spots. There are apps for an iPhone or iPad that use the magnetometer inside these devices (for the compass app) to measure magnetic fields. These EMF-detection apps are not as sophisticated as a professional gauss meter and are limited in the frequency range that they can detect, but they work well to give a general idea of potential problem areas. For the most precision, consult with an EMF inspector to learn which areas of a home or office and what devices are creating the most significant sources of electropollution.

Motor Vehicles

When it comes to vehicles, they all generate significant EMFs but vary in the source of radiation. A 2002 Toyota Corolla measures 10–15 mG at chest level in the driver's seat when idling but pins a gauss meter at more than 100 mG when accelerating. Measurements at groin level in the driver's seat register above 100 mG, while the back seat registers a steady 3 mG, irrespective of whether the car is idling or accelerating. These fields are generated from the alternator of the engine and concentrate on the front and floor areas of motor vehicles.

By contrast, the hybrid 2013 Toyota Prius is much lower overall, measuring 4 mG at groin level of the driver's seat when idling and only increasing to 5 mG with acceleration. At chest height in the driver's seat, the reading drops to 2 mG when idling and 3 mG or less when accelerating. However, the back seat of the Prius registers 6 mG when idling and fluctuates wildly while the car is accelerating, with the gauss meter pinning at more than 100 mG when braking, the phase when the vehicle transfers energy to charge the battery that rests behind the back seats.

What is different with newer vehicles is the addition of an RF field. The 2002 Corolla does not cause any disturbance on an RF meter, but the 2013 Prius emits an 8 second microwave pulse every 6 seconds, around the area of the center dashboard.

An all-electric vehicle, such as the Tesla Model X, fluctuates at 8–9 mG at groin level when in park and increases to 10–15 mG with acceleration. The readings are even less at chest level, registering at only 2–3 mG whether the Model X is moving or not. The floor of the car is where the highest EMF can be detected, originating from the thin but broad battery running along the bottom carriage of the vehicle frame. Whether in the front or back seat, the gauss meter registers more than 100 mG when the Tesla is accelerating or braking and fluctuates between 50 mG and 100 mG when the car is in park but turned on.

The Tesla also emits an RF signal, though it originates from the exterior side view mirrors. Upon measurement, this RF transmission does not account for a significant field strength in the interior. The front windshield of the Tesla contains a special coating that blocks signal transmission from a number of devices, including radiofrequency identification (RFID) transponders used to open electronic gates or pay highway tolls.

Mattresses

A mattress with metal springs can act like an antenna, conducting ambient EMFs around the body while sleeping. In the worst-case scenario, a mattress can become magnetized. This magnetization can be made visible by slowly sliding a compass along the surface of the bed. The needle will twitch every few inches as it passes over a spring due to the offsetting magnetic field being generated by the mattress.

Bed frames should be wood instead of metal, and ideal mattress materials include materials such as natural latex, organic wool, and organic cotton. Mattresses covered in wool have the added benefit of being naturally flame retardant, allowing the manufacturer to sidestep the legal requirement to impregnate toxic flame retardant chemicals into the fabric.

6

REMEDIATION STRATEGIES

Living or working in any building connected to the electrical grid means being exposed to some degree of electropollution. Thankfully, EMFs can be precisely measured and remediated. The solution will depend upon several factors.

If you are in the process of building a home, provisions can be implemented within the design to minimize the impact of 60 Hz EMFs. The best strategy is to have electrical wiring contained within a metal conduit, such as metal-clad (MC) cable instead of plastic-insulated (Romex) wiring. Metal conduit blocks electric (but not magnetic) fields, preventing them from radiating through walls, floors, and ceilings into living spaces. Wiring contained within metal conduit also reduces the impact of voltage transients and other higher-frequency radiation.

Elevated magnetic fields (above 2 mG) also arise from improperly wired circuits if electrical code is not strictly followed. In these instances, the desired direction of current flows over an alternate path, creating an imbalance on multiple circuits. A knowledgeable electrician can measure this by placing a clamp-on ammeter around the cable or circuit in question. These wiring defects often escape detection by home inspectors untrained in the nuances of magnetic field generation.

Another source of aberrant magnetic fields occurs when an electrical current crosses over and flows on metal plumbing pipes, producing what is termed plumbing currents. The resulting magnetic field has the potential to be significant, and the current can be properly measured by an electrician with a clamp-on ammeter. Plumbing currents can be remediated by installation of an insulating coupling (also called a dielectric union) in the water supply line to the building.

Measuring aberrant current as voltage transients is possible with a plug-in electromagnetic interference (EMI) meter designed to register the higher harmonics of 60 Hz AC current in millivolts (mV). Outlets along one circuit will register a similar reading because the current is evenly distributed along the wiring. As multiple circuits become overburdened, the collective electropollution of the building rises, resulting in an increase in voltage transients that may affect nearby buildings. When an EMI meter registers above 100 mV, proceed to one of the following options for remediation.

A favorable decrease in voltage transients can be achieved by removing or unplugging any electrical device that draws current. This includes dimmer switches, variable-speed motors, and device chargers that modulate between DC and AC current.

When possible, dimmer switches should be replaced with a single on-off switch. This may detract from the ambience of a living room but could result in a significant drop in transient voltage. Because dimmer switches contain an electrical part known as a potentiometer (a variable resistor that changes the fraction of current flowing to a device such as a speaker or a light bulb), they generate an additional EMF field via the restriction of voltage.

For lighting, avoid fluorescent bulbs, particularly compact fluorescent lamps (CFLs) that have an electronic ballast built into every bulb. After the inverter rectifies the AC current into DC current, transistors within the CFL ballast convert it into high-frequency AC. This saves a little money on an energy bill over time, but the trade-off is not worth it as these bulbs generate a significant level of transient voltage.

Old-fashioned incandescent bulbs contribute the least to transient voltage, and halogen bulbs are acceptable. LEDs are sometimes problematic but are better than fluorescents. The level of transient voltage created by LED bulbs depends on their construction, something that is not apparent to the average consumer looking at the bulb. With the price of LED bulbs coming down, areas of high usage should be converted to LED lighting if incandescent bulbs are not an option. LEDs last longer than CFLs and don't have the additional problem of containing mercury. If a CFL breaks, open windows and carefully follow mercury-remediation guide-lines.[54]

LED bulbs that screw into 120-volt light receptacles are considerably better than CFLs and generate less transient volt-age. Low-voltage LED lights connected to a dimmer switch and under-counter puck-style LED lights should be avoided as they are prone to generating transient voltage. Small LED bulbs, such as Christmas lights, are generally not problematic.

In general, any bulb connected to or containing an electric ballast tends to produce a high amount of transient voltage. This can be difficult to avoid; many commercial office spaces have tube fluorescent lighting within a drop ceiling. Keeping these lights turned off and using floor lamps improves the situation. If less light is needed, remove two bulbs from a four-bulb receptacle to lower the total demand for current and create less areas for transient voltage to build. A better solution is to have an electrician remove the ballast from overhead lighting receptacles and replace the fluorescent bulbs with LED linear tube bulbs.

Older buildings tend to register more transient voltage, as outdated wiring becomes overloaded by the numerous electrical devices that are plugged in. This is especially true with large power strips occupying multiple outlets along one circuit, as is often the case in offices replete with computers, monitors, phones, and printers as well as home theaters with large-screen TVs and high-wattage speaker systems.

One solution is to hire a skilled electrician trained in EMF remediation to install a kill switch in a room where it is desirable for the power to be turned off at the circuit box, such as the bedroom. This requires the electrician to work with an EMF inspector to test which circuits are affecting the bedroom. The circuits are turned off one by one until the AC fields in the bedroom diminish; those circuits are then tied to the kill switch.

———

Removing sources of transient voltage is the preferred strategy for remediation, however, if outlets are still registering above 100 mV, the next step is to consider installing special outlet filters that draw excess current out of circuits. Available from a few different retailers, special plug-in outlet filters use capacitance to dissipate excess ungrounded current that persists along a circuit as transient voltage. These small white boxes plug in to an electrical outlet, with some models also having a receptacle on the filter so the power from that outlet can continue to be used. Once installed, the drop in transient voltage can immediately be measured on any outlet along the same circuit.

For example, plug an EMI meter into one of four outlets of the same circuit that feeds two walls in a given room. After several moments of fluctuating, the meter will provide an average level of transient voltage in the form of millivolts. Anything above 75 mV is considered unfavorable, but in working with sensitive clients, I like to see the number far below that, into the teens if possible.

Let's say the reading was 850 mV, which is not uncommon. Proceed to a different outlet along that wall, plug in a filter, and see how much the number drops. The number of filters needed to drop the transient voltage to acceptable levels can be precisely measured. For a number as high as 850 mV, this may take four or more filters on the same circuit.

The average circuit in a modern dwelling typically needs one to three filters, however, the more filters that are installed, the less other circuits will require remediation as the total amount of transient voltage decreases. For this reason, when evaluating a building, EMF inspectors will begin by remediating the circuits that are highest behind the walls in spaces occupied for long periods of time.

Outlet filters work best when evenly installed among different electrical circuits. Adding more filters than necessary to suppress transient voltage on one circuit without addressing other circuits has the potential to generate high-frequency magnetic fields. These higher-frequency magnetic emissions appear along the path of the branch circuit from the electric panel out to the room or rooms served and also along the path of power entry into the house. Because EMI meters only measure voltage along wiring, magnetic field generation would be not be detected.

Although getting below 100 mV is a good general guideline, this may not be possible to achieve by simply adding more outlet filters. In cases where transient voltage is entering the house via the power feed from the electrical company, a skilled electrician knowledgeable in EMF mitigation may deem it necessary to install two receptacles (one fed from each phase of the electrical system) adjacent to the electrical service panel, solely for the purpose of installing plug-in line noise filters.

7

SHIELDING STRATEGIES

Avoidance is the best strategy, but what about those instances when that is not possible? I am often asked about different forms of personal protection to shield oneself from the negative effects of EMFs. Many such products exist. Some are intended to be placed around a mobile phone or other device, while others are designed to be worn, such as a pendant. The majority of products in this category seek to block EMF transmission from mobile phones, tablets, and laptops. In some cases, these products act as an EMF-blocking sleeve, enveloping a mobile phone or tablet when not in use. They work by cutting off all signal transmission as if the device were shut off. Other products are designed to form a physical barrier between the device and the body, such as a pad placed under a laptop when using it on one's lap.

Some larger shielding devices can indeed provide a measurable decrease in EMFs by blocking electrical fields, but they don't block magnetic fields. As such, these products can only mitigate half the problem; however, that effect is desirable and worth consideration for someone surrounded by these devices for long periods every day.

Of the devices where shielding is a consideration, mobile phones are the worst offenders as they emit both microwave radiation (when not in airplane mode) as well as lower-level EMFs produced by any electrical device. This is also true for tablets enabled with cellular service.

Laptops, tablets, and devices operating with only Wi-Fi don't spike an RF meter quite as much, but they still produce a strong field of electropollution within a few inches of the device, affecting the hands as one types, clicks, or holds the device.

E-readers without a backlit screen emit the least electropollution given the small battery and low power usage. These older devices only use Wi-Fi when downloading a book, so the Wi-Fi can be shut off for the majority of their use. Newer e-reader models with a backlit screen are equivalent to tablets both in functionality and EMF output.

Shielding Products

There are differences in how shielding devices work.

Products like Brink cases do not block RF fields so much as direct them away from the user (as much as 67%, according to their website). This is most relevant for a mobile phone that is held to the head. Brink product testing reliably measures a decrease in—not elimination of—the RF field at the front of the device but an increase in the RF field toward the back.

It is a compromise worth considering given the preference to protect the delicate neurocircuitry of the brain. Those who are highly sensitive to EMFs may still notice numbness or a buzzing sensation in the hands that travels up the arms.

The manufacturers of DefenderShield and SafeSleeve also report a measurable decrease in EMFs between the user and device, like a wall blocking all transmission along one spatial plane. These devices are only effective at protecting the area of the body where a tablet or laptop rests. Although they provide a modicum of protection to the vital and reproductive organs if the devices are used while lounging on the couch, EMFs will still course upward to the head and outward into the hands, a contributing risk factor for conditions such as chronic headaches and carpal tunnel syndrome.

Both of these companies offer a product to encase a mobile phone, dampening the transmission of EMFs while not in use, again along one spatial plane. This works to shield an individual from the device when carried in a pocket or held to the head but offers no protection to the hand holding the phone. These shielding devices don't block both sides of a mobile phone as that would inhibit the reception of calls and text messages, a testament to their efficacy that also highlights their limitations.

Personal Protection Products

There are many nonshielding products that claim to modulate EMF signals and render them harmless to the user when worn or affixed to devices such as mobile phones. These smaller, charm-like products simply do not stand up to measurable scrutiny when placed between a source of EMF and the appropriate meter.

The manufacturers advertise that benefits can be "felt" or shown through muscle testing or various forms of dowsing. Although I am open to the use of these techniques by skilled practitioners, the skeptic in me is concerned about confirmation bias that feeds marketing hype. We have objective tools to measure the effectiveness of these products, so the healthy skeptic should question any protection claim that cannot be individually and repeatably tested.

Furthermore, just because an EMF-protection product claims the user will feel an increased sense of well-being doesn't mean the environment has changed. Painkillers help people feel better too but do nothing to mitigate the underlying cause of pain. Radon, mold, carbon monoxide—the toxicity of these harmful environmental exposures may go undetected, yet their pernicious influence persists. EMFs are no different in this regard.

For those who feel a difference using these products, the most obvious explanation is the power of expectation generating a placebo effect. This is a valid phenomenon and should not be altogether dismissed. The power of the mind is well-known to lower pain and stress hormones. It is therefore absolutely possible to subjectively feel better about EMF exposure through use of these products while still objectively exposing the body to harmful levels of radiation. If this false sense of security comes at the expense of properly avoiding, remediating, or shielding EMF radiation, little else has been achieved beyond masking the problem.

Grounding Products

Various products designed to connect a device or the user to the ground plug of an outlet have entered the marketplace. The products that attach a grounding strap to a person are purported to work by discharging static charge built up from electrical devices while supplying a steady stream of negative ions, as would occur if one stands barefoot on the surface of the Earth. The documented health benefits of grounding are attributed to the absorption of negative ions through the skin that quench positively charged free radicals.[55]

There is some controversy surrounding products that connect an individual with a grounding cord and strap to the ground plug of an outlet. For starters, they provide no benefit if the circuit itself is not properly grounded. This is at least quickly and inexpensively tested with an outlet checker, available at hardware stores.

More concerning, connecting an individual to a ground plug of an overcharged circuit may increase total body voltage rather than dissipate it. As the grounding circuit of an outlet can carry electrical noise, determining the efficacy of these products requires careful testing with an oscilloscope to measure the change in millivolts when connected to the ground plug of an electrical outlet.

Supporters of grounding to an outlet cite the use of a voltmeter to measure a decrease in electrical potential when grounding (to match that of the Earth) as evidence of safety. However, a drop in electrical potential does not assume the current is bouncing off the individual as if the person were in a Faraday cage. Rather, the current flows through highly conductive human tissue on its way to reaching near-zero electrical potential via the ground.

There may be circumstances when grounding to an electrical outlet may be safe and beneficial,[56] but this does not appear to be categorically true. The safest method of grounding is to walk barefoot on wet grass or a sandy beach.

A less risky indoor option is to attach grounding cords to devices that generate an AC electric field but do not have a ground prong on the plug of the power adapter. Laptops and computers that either operate on battery power or are plugged in with a two-prong power adapter can be grounded by a special ground plug connected to a standard USB plug. The USB plug contacts the metal structure of the hardware and conducts the electrical potential away from the user.

A grounding strategy to address the charge built up while driving is a static strap designed to connect to the chassis of a motor vehicle. Install these conductive straps toward the center of the undercarriage to prevent concerned observers from repeatedly notifying the driver that something is hanging off the car.

8

CONNECTING THE RESEARCH DOTS

In perhaps the most compelling and landmark study to date, the U.S. Department of Health and Human Services National Toxicology Program (NTP) issued a press release in November of 2018 with the results of a peer review process of research on mobile phone RF radiation conducted in 2016. The panel of 11 experts reexamined the data based on the NTP's scale of decreasing risk: clear evidence, some evidence, equivocal evidence, and no evidence. By their criteria, equivocal evidence of carcinogenic activity "is demonstrated by studies that are interpreted as showing a marginal increase of neoplasms that may be chemically related."[57]

In one report on mice that were exposed to CDMA- or GSM-modulated cellphone RF in the 1,900 MHz range, the panel agreed with the findings of the 2016 research. The panel concluded that there was "equivocal evidence" of carcinogenic activity in male mice for the combined incidences of fibrosarcoma, sarcoma, or malignant fibrous histiocytoma in the skin, incidences of alveolar/bronchiolar adenoma or

carcinoma (combined) in the lung, and incidences of hepato-
blastoma of the liver.

For female mice, there was "equivocal evidence" of
carcinogenic activity in incidences of malignant lymphoma
(all organs).[58]

In a second report, rats were exposed to regular intervals
of either CDMA or GSM-modulated cellphone RF of 900
MHz, in some cases for up to two years. Initial data showed
that of the eight cohorts studied, five showed "equivocal
evidence" while two showed "some evidence" of carcinogenic
activity. Only in one cohort could researchers confidently
conclude that there was "no evidence" of carcinogenic
activity.[59]

Their initial assessment alone should be sufficient to give
pause and seriously consider the health consequences of
EMFs. However, upon review of the data by the panel, the
conclusions became more concerning, now with recommendations to upgrade five cohorts to "some evidence" or "clear
evidence" of carcinogenic activity:

- For male rats exposed to GSM-modulated
  cellphone RF radiation, malignant schwannoma in
  the heart was reclassified from "some evidence" to
  "clear evidence" of carcinogenic activity.
  Malignant glioma of the brain was reclassified
  from "equivocal evidence" to "some evidence" of
  carcinogenic activity. Pheochromocytoma, a tumor
  in the adrenal gland, was reclassified from
  "equivocal evidence" to "some evidence" of
  carcinogenic activity.
- For female rats exposed to GSM-modulated

cellphone RF radiation, malignant schwannoma of the heart was reclassified from "no evidence" to "equivocal evidence" of carcinogenic activity.

- For male rats exposed to CDMA-modulated cellphone RF radiation, malignant schwannoma in the heart was reclassified from "some evidence" to "clear evidence" of carcinogenic activity. Malignant glioma of the brain was reclassified from "equivocal evidence" to "some evidence" of carcinogenic activity.
- For female rats exposed to CDMA-modulated cellphone RF radiation, malignant schwannoma in the heart was reclassified from "no evidence" to "equivocal evidence" of carcinogenic activity.[60]

Overall this research details a disturbing trend. In no case was the evidence downgraded to suggest a decreased risk of cancer compared to the original findings. Animal studies are not the only line of evidence suggesting an association between cancer and EMFs. On the contrary, we now have four corroborating lines of evidence demonstrating EMFs are a far more significant risk factor than previously thought for the development of a number of cancers.

1. **Carlo's pioneering work on the WTR project:** This research showed conclusively that EMFs cause genetic damage by measuring the presence of micronuclei in living cells exposed to RF radiation. We can no longer equate safety with

industry standards of SAR ratings for mobile phones based on thermal output. Biological damage from exposure to RF radiation has been confirmed at levels that do not markedly heat underlying tissue.

2. **Research elucidating plausible mechanisms:** To explain a novel biological effect as Carlo has reported, a corresponding model must be presented to the scientific community for scrutiny. Pall's work confirming cell damage from EMFs through tissue calcium changes is the key that opens the door to a plausible mechanism for what Carlo's team and others have observed in micronuclei experiments. Add to Pall's work a growing body of research uncovering additional mechanisms of immune dysregulation from EMFs, chief among them being suppression of melatonin production. We now have multiple pieces of evidence implicating a broad range of EMF frequencies with biological damage.

3. **Epidemiological evidence linking EMF exposure to cancer:** Epidemiological evidence shows an increase in a number of human cancers following long-term exposure to several EMFs, including mobile phone RF radiation, voltage transients, and the ELF EMFs of modern electrification. Much of that research in relation to cancer is discussed in this book; a broader compilation of research on the health effects of EMFs can be found in the 2012 BioInitiative Report.[61]

4. **NTP research showing "clear evidence" of increased cancer growth from RF radiation in animal models:** As detailed above, by comparing RF radiation-exposed rats with a cohort of control unexposed rats, NTP studies experimentally clarify the cancer link. Since we cannot ethically expose humans to tantamount lab conditions, we must connect the dots between the experimental animal studies and epidemiological evidence in humans. The work of Carlo and Pall connects those dots, taking us from effects observed in a lab to real-world consequences.

Perhaps you are beginning to feel like a lab rat yourself? There is the temptation to stick one's head in the sand when collectively viewing these lines of evidence. It is my hope that the strategies detailed in the last four chapters will provide the fuel to begin your journey toward a healthier relationship with technology.

CONCLUSION

"It is no measure of good health to be well-adjusted to a profoundly sick society."

—Jiddu Krishnamurti, philosopher

───────

The animal studies from the NTP research showing "clear evidence" of increased cancer growth from RF radiation should be enough for a critical reexamination of our relationship with radiation-emitting technology.

For someone with a cancer diagnosis, **any** evidence of carcinogenic activity is concerning. Even equivocal evidence is far from comforting. Until long-term human studies (that so far have shown the opposite) can claim no evidence of carcinogenic activity, the precautionary principle must be vigorously applied.

We have every right to be cautious, living in a modern world plagued with chronic degenerative disease. Statistics posted by the American Cancer Society on cancer incidence for the United States from 2012 through 2014 indicate that 1 in 3 people will develop cancer.[62] By some estimates, that number may grow to be as epidemic as 1 in 2 people in places like the United Kingdom.[63]

We are facing a dilemma in which our genetics are loading the gun and radiation-emitting technology is pulling the trigger. That's not to say that technological innovation is inherently harmful, but we must now consider how that innovation is impacting our health. We are simply unable to predict the future and tend to do a poor job objectifying data when a paycheck is on the line. We are also a species vulnerable to addictions, with personal electronic devices being the latest human pacifier.

We assuage our academic blind spots with the power of hindsight but fail to use the wisdom gleaned to act with caution in foresight. It is this manner of cognitive bias that perpetuated the decades-long myth that dietary saturated fats cause heart disease.[64]

Even when science draws statistically significant associations, rarely does it change our behavior when short-term gain and addiction cloud our judgment. A history of cigarette smoking is unquestionably the single largest risk factor for lung cancer, yet many still choose to puff toward a future of black, tarnished lungs.

Most cancers do not have as predictable a causative link as smoking does for the lungs. With so many different types of cancer and environmental stressors, it is difficult, if not impossible, to rectify each individual's susceptibility (genetic) with the unique combination of environmental triggers (epigenetic) that will manifest as a cancer diagnosis.

In the absence of artificial intelligence driving a global algorithm of cancer risk factors, we are left with leading science to present data points; common sense connects the research into reasonable positions on adopting new technology and actionable steps to decrease risk.

Anecdotally, the minority of the population who claim to be electrosensitive are akin to those individuals who become acutely ill breathing cigarette smoke. We can dismiss these technophobes as eccentric Luddites, but are they the few registering the acute toxicity that belies the chronic disease lurking in the shadows?

On the contrary, it is unlikely that the research presented here will persuade the technophile who concludes the issue is overstated and the rhetoric melodramatic. This individual is akin to the addicted smoker who refuses to quit despite a hacking cough and yearly bronchitis. There will always be patients with emphysema who choose to keep smoking as well as brain cancer patients who take the oncologist's call on a mobile phone, answering it on the affected side.

Like the varied effects of nicotine, there is the good with the bad. Nicotine is arguably one of the best nootropics (smart drugs) when delivered to the exclusion of the combustion byproducts accompanying its smoked form.

The wireless revolution has its conveniences, like when we adjust a home thermostat from a smartphone before arriving home from vacation. In either case, we must weigh the benefits against the risks and carefully decide what level of technology we allow into our homes and lives.

If you have been diagnosed with cancer or are taking proactive steps to prevent cancer, you must adopt the right frame of mind in your deliberations. The question is no longer if or even how EMFs cause cancer growth. Rather, to what extent for each individual, given the many carcinogenic risk factors to which we are all exposed, does the environment promote cancer? Research may eventually reveal that some people are genetically predisposed to cancer development when exposed to EMFs but not before multiple generations are subjected to this mass experiment.

Moreover, many of us are becoming increasingly reliant on technology, in some cases to the point of addiction. Like cigarettes, technological addiction is chemical in nature as well as psychological. With every compulsive check of email or social media, a little hit of the satisfaction-inducing neurotransmitter dopamine gets released in the brain.[65] The modulation of dopamine from technological addiction might not be as immediately potent as nicotine's effects, but it adds to the psychological burden of an irradiated world replete with addictions and distractions.

Simply designating a behavior as destructive does not guarantee behavior change on a large scale, nor does listing off compelling research studies. Sometimes it takes a scare to be roused from the illusion, waking in shock to find more and more people being diagnosed with cancer.

I was scared when diagnosed with stage 4 cancer at the age of 34. Questioning the status quo, I contemplated the larger story that is the cancer epidemic and did not like what I saw. There is a world of risk factors bombarding our bodies and hijacking our ability to live healthy and happy lives.

Perhaps EMF exposure is a drop in the bucket in a world swimming in a chemical sea of carcinogens, but I predict time will expose EMFs to be as significant a carcinogenic factor as smoking. With vested interests poised in a lockstep march into an increasingly technological world, it is up to you, the individual, to exercise caution and safeguard the health and well-being of your family.

AFTERWORD—BY CHARLES KEEN

Brandon LaGreca has done an extraordinary job of articulating the science underlying the EMF health effects issue, the different types of EMFs that are ubiquitous in our world, and the many steps that we can take to begin cleaning up our electromagnetic environment. There is indeed much that can be done just based on the information in this book, yet there are many EMF problems that cannot be perceived or even predicted. We must use the tools of the trade to find them or call upon a qualified EMF inspector, testing person, or consultant to examine our homes and offices, and provide guidance in mitigating any problems that show up.

Hiring an EMF Testing Provider

Finding a qualified EMF testing person could be a challenge, depending on where you live. An online search for terms like "EMF testing," "EMF consultant," or "EMF inspector" is likely to produce a confusing array of irrelevant results along with a few good people, most of whom are very far away. With a little searching, you can find two or three lists of EMF consultants across the United States and Canada. Although inclusion on a list does not imply that a provider is competent or qualified, it is a good start and the lists are worth perusing to see if there is anyone near you. If you are lucky enough to find someone, the next step is to check that person out, and a few suggestions are coming up.

One organization that maintains such a list is **The International Institute for Building-Biology & Ecology**. This group operates a training program focused on creation of healthy homes and workplaces, and EMF is one component of their broader environmental curriculum. Students who complete the basic program and take some advanced courses can acquire certification as an Electromagnetic Radiation Specialist, a credential you definitely want to check for on the list. It is essential to understand that capabilities vary widely depending upon extent of training and how long someone has been practicing. As in most fields of work, experience is by far the best teacher.

Just as being on a list does not confirm that a person is qualified, not being present on a list certainly does not mean that a person is unqualified. Some people who are active in the EMF world have taken a more traditional academic path, or have transitioned from a related career as a health professional or an electrician. There is a strong base of EMF knowledge and experience among these professionals who operate independently of any organization.

Once you have found a reasonably close person or company that looks promising, it's time to call them up. A few easy questions will help you determine if this person can meet your needs, and will also guide the testing provider in describing what he or she does and how they can help you. You could start by explaining that you are interested in having your home tested for EMFs. This is often called an EMF survey. If you're considering purchase or rental of a property and want to make sure there are no unforeseen problems, that is called a pre-purchase EMF inspection, an extremely important step before signing a contract!

Here are some questions you may want to ask a prospective service provider, but keep in mind that not everyone is going to have the most impressive background or the greatest experience or all the perfect answers. That's not really necessary. If what they tell you sounds reasonable and is consistent with what you have read in this book and gives you the sense that they are operating with integrity, it will probably turn out fine.

1) What kind of training have you had?

Formal training from some reputable organization is always best, unless the person already has a degree or certificate in a closely related field and a good amount of experience with EMFs. Most people in the business will be able to explain their background sufficiently for you to understand their qualifications. It is unfortunate, but there are no required training programs, national standards, or certifications for people who perform EMF testing, only voluntary ones.

2) How long have you been working in this field?

Training and experience are both important in the development of professional capability, but an abundance of one can make up for a lack of the other. For example, a new entrant to the EMF-testing business who has had solid training and received some type of relevant certification should be completely capable of performing basic EMF testing. More senior people with lots of experience are always available to advise new entrants to this field, so there is a deeper store of knowledge that can be drawn upon as needed.

3) What types of EMF can you test for?

All legitimate EMF providers should be able to test for AC magnetic fields, AC electric fields, and RF fields. Many can also test for transient voltage or dirty electricity.

4) What is the cost of a home EMF survey, and about how long does it take?

The answer to this question will depend on size and complexity of the area to be tested. For example, is it a small apartment or a large custom home? Most providers scale their fees to size, driving distance, things to be tested, and sometimes the type of report that a customer requires. They should be able to quote a firm price at the time arrangements are made, before coming out to your location.

Avoid These Testing Providers

1) Anyone whose website is more focused on instilling fear than on educating you and explaining the services that are offered:

There are some providers who try to make you even more fearful about EMF than you may already be, for their own benefit. Fear-mongering is destructive and exploitative, and there is absolutely no place for it in any legitimate business. There is also at least one company who states on its website that using an EMF meter on your own is so hazardous that you risk electrocution, death, or other serious harm—a profoundly ridiculous assertion. Fortunately, recognizing outlandish claims and shameless self-aggrandizement is not too difficult for most of us. Awareness of a problem followed by action toward a solution is all that is ever required.

2) People who purport to provide EMF-testing services, but who in reality are focused exclusively on dirty electricity testing and abatement:

These people are unable or reluctant to test for the full range of EMF parameters discussed in this book, and their primary solution for EMFs is to install plug-in filters throughout the house. There are not many of these people but they are out there. The questions above about training and what types of EMFs one can test for will help you avoid this disappointing and very limited service offering.

3) Large magnetic-shielding companies that serve commercial clients and RF testing companies that serve the telecom or broadcast industries:

Although some of these companies may offer to perform residential testing, they are generally unaware of the EMF levels that are relevant to customers who are approaching the exposure issue from a precautionary standpoint.

4) Home inspectors who mainly perform structural building inspections but offer EMF testing as an add-on service or sideline business:

Consider this option only when you have contracted for a standard pre-purchase home inspection in an area where there are no full-time EMF-testing people available.

Self-Testing for EMFs

The unfortunate reality is that in many parts of the country there are no legitimate testing providers within a reasonable driving distance. Most states don't even have a single EMF consultant, qualified or not! This includes some very major cities. Much of the East and West coasts are covered and part of the Great Lakes region, but the interior of the country is not. Residential services are inherently price-limited, and except for rare cases that price precludes air travel. So what is one to do?

Many people will choose to purchase a good consumer-grade EMF meter (or two or three) and do their own testing. If you buy the right meter it is really quite easy, and fun! Your eyes will be opened to an electromagnetic world that our normal human senses cannot perceive but which has been explained, measured, and manipulated by physicists and engineers for many decades. The instruments simply pick up where our eyes and ears leave off. But the operative phrase is "the right meter." The market is populated by countless EMF instruments ranging in price from a few dollars to a few thousand dollars. Most of the low end of that range is pure junk and will lead you into a dark place of confusion or unwarranted concern. The high-end instruments are exclusively for professionals and present a level of complexity unsuitable for beginning users. Guidance in selecting an appropriate meter, and suggestions drawn from user experience, are presented in the sections below.

The only real drawback to self-testing will become apparent if you discover EMF levels that are clearly elevated and you have no idea what to do about it. That would be the time to seek out professional assistance, even if the only providers are distant from you. Some EMF specialists offer distance consultation by phone on a paid basis, so there is often a good solution only a phone call away.

Magnetic Field Testing

This is arguably the most important type of EMF to test for, as the science supporting adverse health effects is the most extensive, especially where cancer is concerned. Magnetic field measurements are easily performed with an instrument called an AC gaussmeter. A 3-axis (non-directional) meter is essential to avoid the difficulty and errors that always occur when an inexperienced person tries to use an inexpensive

1-axis meter. Most gaussmeters sold in North America read out in units of mG (milligauss). Residential levels are typically less than 1 mG unless there is a power line nearby, a problem with mis-wired electrical circuits in the house, or current on the water pipes.

The best testing procedure is to walk slowly through the house while watching the meter for any "hot spots." Take readings where people are normally present, and turn lights on and off to see if the readings change dramatically (they should not). Avoid holding the meter right up against a wall or near an electrical device, as readings in those locations can be misleading.

If a power line is the suspected magnetic field source, the measured level will change substantially as load on the electric company's distribution system changes, so it's advisable to take readings at different times of the day and under different weather conditions to observe the range of numbers that will exist at a given location.

The best choice for an economically priced 3-axis gaussmeter is the **TriField TF2**. It is easy to use, and when set on the Standard Magnetic scale (not the Weighted scale), the readings are accurate enough for any non-professional use.

Electric Field Testing

AC electric fields arise from any unshielded electrical wire or power line and are present whenever the circuit is live. Wiring in the walls, ceiling, and floor of most single-family homes and some smaller apartment buildings is unshielded, plastic-covered cable, so people are exposed continuously to this type of EMF. Electric field measurements are performed with an instrument called an electric field meter (How simple is that?) and expressed in units of V/m (Volts per meter).

Many people who have studied the issue feel that electric field exposure is most significant during sleep, so the main focus for measurements should be the bedroom, especially at the headboard. This is usually the point nearest the wall and also nearest the electrical cords from bedside lights plugged into a receptacle. Most AC electric field meters are not very sensitive, so in a sleeping area it is desirable to see numbers near the lowest that the meter will read, preferably 1 V/m or less.

The **TriField TF2** recommended above is also the best choice for an economically priced electric field meter. It should be used on the Standard Electric scale.

Radio Frequency Testing

RF is one of the big EMF issues that you will want to test for, yet it is the most challenging. There are a number of reasons for this: (a) Many different measurement units are in use, most of which appear as cryptic and indecipherable combinations of letters and numbers; (b) the readout on an RF meter jumps around a lot and appears unstable; (c) some meters have multiple settings to figure out; and (d) all decent RF meters cost more than other types of EMF meter.

But do not be intimidated! You can do this, and we will guide you through it. Upon completion, you can bask in the satisfaction of having learned to do something of real value, and you didn't have to pay anyone else to do it for you.

First, get to know your RF meter by reading the manual. It will be time well-spent even though everything will not be immediately clear.

RF levels are best measured while standing stationary rather than walking around. You simply take a reading at each place of interest where people are routinely present and write it down on a notepad. For accurate readings with most RF meters, you should hold the meter upright with the presumed signal source in front of you—that is, with the signal coming toward the back of the meter. If you are not sure where the signal is coming from, turn around slowly until you see the highest reading. Avoid holding the meter near a wall because the reading could be erroneous due to the presence of electrical wiring or metal studs.

If you are using the meter we recommend below, there will be two numbers: a peak reading and an average reading. They are expressed in different units, as shown on the face of the meter. As you watch the meter, the numbers on the display will be jumping around and the lights will be moving up and down. For our purposes, the two rows of lights will provide the easiest reading. Watch for the highest light that consistently appears, ignoring very occasional flashes of a higher light. Do this for the left row of lights and write down the peak reading; then do it for the right row and write down the average reading. That's it, and you can move on to the next measurement point.

There is an interesting observation that you can make with this instrument because it is reading peak and average at the same time. If the lights on the left side are consistently reaching a higher position than the lights on the right side, the signal you are measuring has a more pulsed character, such as from a WiFi router. It is thought that such highly pulsed signals may be more biologically active and thus worthy of greater attention than a non-pulsed signal.

You will notice that we are measuring in units of V/m (Volts per meter) and $\mu W/m^2$ (microWatts per meter squared). These are the preferred and most common units. There are around 10 other RF measurement units that you will encounter with other instruments and in some documents about RF exposure, and those units can all be converted back and forth from one to the other. Unless you are an engineer with a real need to know, don't worry about all this confusion and let it pass by without a second thought.

Knowing the source of the RF signal you are measuring is important, so be aware of nearby sources such as WiFi routers or cordless home phones that are running all the time. Many people who are initially concerned about cell towers or smart meters find that their own in-building devices are by far the dominant exposure source. You will certainly want to observe how much they contribute to your indoor environment, but be prepared to turn them off if you are trying to measure the signals from something outside like a cell tower. Your own cell phone will also produce signals sporadically even when a call is not in progress, so airplane mode is a good idea while testing.

The RF meter that we recommend, as well as many others on the market, will not measure signals from AM or FM radio towers. So you will need to determine through other means (such as your eyes) if there are any very close, like less than a mile.

The best consumer-grade RF meter available is the **Acoustimeter AM-10**, which strikes a perfect balance between performance and simplicity. It is sensitive, accurate, easy to use (only one on/off switch), covers a broad frequency range, and reads out in the most commonly used units. Best of all, it lets you hear a representation of what you are measuring to assist in source identification. (You will not hear the voice audio of signals from cell phones or towers, just the sound of digital signals, which you will soon learn to recognize.)

Transient Voltage Testing

Brandon has already presented a good explanation of this, and that will get you started. Transient voltage (dirty electricity) testing and remediation is an evolving science, and there are still open questions about the best approach to deal with the transient voltage that is always present to some extent on electrical wiring. As with most types of EMF, it's always wise to be aware of new studies that may emerge, and which could alter the recommendations that we currently follow.

The best meter choice is the **Greenwave Broadband EMI Meter**, because it reads out in mV (milliVolts), a standard scientific unit, and covers a wider frequency range than most other meters. It also lets you hear the electrical noise on the wiring in your house, which is not only a very cool feature, but often a great help in identifying the noisy electrical devices that produce high readings.

———

It can be deeply disconcerting to many people to learn that we are exposed to so many EMFs from so many sources, but you can take great comfort in knowing that most elevated EMF conditions are fully correctable once you find out about them and bring into play the proper resources. But it is still the responsibility of each individual to become aware of their electromagnetic environment and to act upon what they know.

Thanks for reading.

If you have benefited from this book, please share it with others and leave a review on Amazon to help spread awareness to the cancer community.

Visit www.EmpoweredPatientBlog.com to learn more about Brandon's journey. You can also sign up for his newsletter to receive blog updates and news about future book releases.

Join the conversation and share your story on our Facebook page,www.Facebook.com/EmpoweredPatientBlog. Together we will grow stronger through and beyond cancer.

ACKNOWLEDGMENTS

I wish to express my gratitude to those who have enhanced the manuscript for this book. Many thanks to Joy Hernes for providing a layperson's perspective, Marcin Baranowski for science editing and sketching out the early design for a book cover, and Mary Cordaro for her sage advice as a practitioner of Building Biology.

A hearty thanks to Charles Keen for offering his substantial expertise in EMF inspection and remediation. Through our conversations over the finer details of the manuscript, it became clear that he was the ideal person to write the afterword, for which I am exceedingly grateful.

Finally, a sincere thanks to Cindy Berg for being my consummate copyediting champion. Whenever someone claims I'm a good writer, I respond that I have a great editor.

This book was crowdfunded with generous support of many family members, friends, and patients. Thank you all for getting the literary ball rolling; there will be more.

ABOUT BRANDON LAGRECA

Brandon LaGreca, LAc, MAcOM, is a 2005 graduate of the Oregon College of Oriental Medicine, a licensed acupuncturist in the state of Wisconsin, and nationally certified in the practice of Oriental medicine.

Having been exposed to acupuncture at a young age, Brandon began his formal study of traditional Chinese medicine through the practice of qi gong at age 13. After the completion of his master's degree in acupuncture and Oriental medicine, he continued his education with postgraduate clinical work in Nanjing, China.

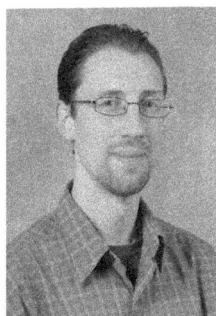

Photo by Andrew Seiden

In 2015, Brandon was diagnosed with stage 4 non-Hodgkin's lymphoma. He achieved full remission eight months later by following an integrative medicine protocol that included immunotherapy without the use of chemotherapy, radiation, or surgery.

Brandon created his *Empowered Patient Blog* to share his experience growing stronger through and beyond cancer. He now lectures and writes extensively on holistic cancer therapies and is a columnist for *Acupuncture Today*.

As the founder and director of East Troy Acupuncture, an integrative medical clinic serving southeast Wisconsin, Brandon specializes in whole food nutrition, ancestral health, and environmental medicine.

facebook.com/EmpoweredPatientBlog

ABOUT CHARLES KEEN

Charles Keen has been professionally involved in EMF-related activities since 1992. His background prior to that time spanned nearly two decades in the telecommunications industry, in a range of technical, engineering, and management positions that included development of test procedures for RF communications systems.

Keen is a member of, and certified by, the International Association of Electrical Inspectors. He holds a bachelor's degree from the University of Maryland, where his training focused on environmental health, occupational safety, and risk analysis. Keen has presented for a number of real estate, inspection, and school groups and was featured in an article by *The Washington Post* about the public perception of the risk of magnetic fields near power lines.

He is the developer of active magnetic shielding equipment for reduction of power line EMFs and primarily focuses on site-specific active shielding system design, RF site assessment and analysis, and EMI problem resolution.

Through his company, EMF Services LLC, Keen provides electromagnetic field testing and remediation to clients worldwide. Since 1992, the company has conducted survey and mitigation projects for commercial clients, city and county governments, the U.S. government, public and private schools, property developers, apartment complexes, and several hundred residential customers.

EMF Services regularly conducts full-scale mitigation projects, including the installation of active magnetic shielding systems and wiring revisions to achieve National Electrical Code compliance. The EMF Services team feels that an objective scientific approach to this issue, along with proven technological intervention strategies, offers the best opportunity to move beyond the misinformation that has characterized public discussion of EMFs.

REFERENCES

1. McCarty, David E., et al. "Electromagnetic Hypersensitivity: Evidence for a Novel Neurological Syndrome." International Journal of Neuroscience, vol. 121, no. 12, Nov. 2011, pp. 670–76. Crossref, doi: 10.3109/00207454.2011.608139

2. Federal Communications Commission. "Wireless Devices and Health Concerns." 26 May 2011. https://www.fcc.gov/consumers/guides/wireless-devices-and-health-concerns. (accessed 24 August 2018).

3. Gandhi, Om P., et al. "Exposure Limits: The Underestimation of Absorbed Cell Phone Radiation, Especially in Children." Electromagnetic Biology and Medicine, vol. 31, no. 1, Mar. 2012, pp. 34–51. Crossref, doi: 10.3109/15368378.2011.622827

4. Schmid, Gernot, and Niels Kuster. "The Discrepancy between Maximum in Vitro Exposure Levels and Realistic Conservative Exposure Levels of Mobile Phones Operating at 900/1800 MHz: In Vitro Versus Real Mobile Phone Exposure." Bioelectromagnetics, vol. 36, no. 2, Feb. 2015, pp. 133–48. Crossref, doi: 10.1002/bem.21895

5. Environmental Health Trust. "Cell Phone Wireless Radiation Litigation." https://ehtrust.org/key-issues/cell-phone-radiation-litigation/ (accessed 26 November 2018).

6. International Agency for Research on Cancer. "IARC Classifies Radiofrequency Electromagnetic Fields as Possibly Carcinogenic to Humans." 31 May 2011, www.iarc.fr/en/media-centre/pr/2011/pdfs/pr208_E.pdf. (accessed 12 July 2018).

7. The INTERPHONE Study Group. "Brain Tumour Risk in Relation to Mobile Telephone Use: Results of the INTERPHONE International Case-Control Study." International Journal of Epidemiology, vol. 39, no. 3, June 2010, pp. 675–94. Crossref, doi: 10.1093/ije/dyq079

8. Hardell, L., et al. "Long-term Use of Cellular Phones and Brain Tumours: Increased Risk Associated with Use for >=10 Years." Occupational and Environmental Medicine, vol. 64, no. 9, Jan. 2007, pp. 626–32. Crossref, doi: 10.1136/oem.2006.029751

9. Khurana, Vini G., et al. "Cell Phones and Brain Tumors: A Review Including the Long-Term Epidemiologic Data." Surgical Neurology, vol. 72, no. 3, Sept. 2009, pp. 205–14. Crossref, doi: 10.1016/j.surneu.2009.01.019

10. Bortkiewicz, Alicja, et al. "Mobile Phone Use and Risk for Intracranial Tumors and Salivary Gland Tumors—A Meta-Analysis." International Journal of Occupational Medicine and Environmental Health, Feb. 2017. Crossref, doi: 10.13075/ijomeh.1896.00802

11. Cardis, E., et al. "Risk of Brain Tumours in Relation to Estimated RF Dose from Mobile Phones: Results from Five Interphone Countries." Occupational and Environmental Medicine, vol. 68, no. 9, Sept. 2011, pp. 631–40. Crossref, doi: 10.1136/oemed-2011-100155

12. Hepworth, Sarah J., et al. "Mobile Phone Use and Risk of Glioma in Adults: Case-Control Study." BMJ, vol. 332, no. 7546, Apr. 2006, pp. 883–87. Crossref, doi: 10.1136/bmj.38720.687975.55

13. "What You Need to Know about the New Study on Cellphones and Cancer." PBS NewsHour, 28 May 2016, https://www.pbs.org/newshour/science/what-you-need-to-know-about-the-new-study-on-cellphones-and-cancer. (accessed 12 July 2018).

14. McVicar, Nancy. "With So Many Different Findings from Cell-Phone Studies, Experts Say It Is Difficult to Get Clear Answers on Health Risks." Sun-Sentinel.com, http://www. sun-sentinel.com/sfl-oresearch02oct02-story.html. (accessed 12 July 2018).

15. Huss, Anke, et al. "Source of Funding and Results of Studies of Health Effects of Mobile Phone Use: Systematic Review of Experimental Studies." Environmental Health Perspectives, vol. 115, no. 1, Sept. 2006, pp. 1–4. Crossref, doi: 10.1289%2Fehp.9149

16. Hertsgaard, Mark, and Mark Dowie. "How Big Wireless Made Us Think that Cell Phones Are Safe: A Special Investigation." The Nation, 29 March 2018, http://www.thenation. com/article/how-big-wireless-made-us-think-that-cell-phones-are-safe-a-special-investigation/. (accessed 12 July 2018).

17. Tice, Raymond R., et al. "Genotoxicity of Radiofrequency Signals. I. Investigation of DNA Damage and Micronuclei Induction in Cultured Human Blood Cells." Bioelectromagnetics, vol. 23, no. 2, Feb. 2002, pp. 113–26. Crossref, doi: 10.1002/bem.104

18. Bisht, Kheem S., et al. "Chromosome Damage and Micronucleus Formation in Human Blood Lymphocytes Exposed In Vitro to Radiofrequency Radiation at a Cellular Telephone Frequency (847.74 MHz, CDMA)." Radiation Research, vol. 156, no. 4, Oct. 2001, pp. 430–32. Crossref, doi: 10.1667/0033-7587(2001)156[0430:CDAMFI]2.0.CO;2

19. Persson, B.R., Salford, L.G. & Brun, A. "Blood-Brain Barrier Permeability in Rats Exposed to Electromagnetic Fields Used in Wireless Communication." Wireless Networks (1997) 3: 455. Crossref, doi: 10.1023/A:1019150510840

20. Gustavino, Bianca, et al. "Exposure to 915 MHz Radiation Induces Micronuclei in *Vicia Faba* Root Tips." Mutagenesis, vol. 31, no. 2, Mar. 2016, pp. 187–92. Crossref, doi: 10.1093/mutage/gev071

21. Hallberg, Örjan. "Cancer Incidence vs. FM Radio Transmitter Density." Electromagnetic Biology and Medicine, vol. 35, no. 4, Oct. 2016, pp. 343–47. Crossref, doi: 10.3109/15368378.2016.1138122

22. Hallberg, Örjan, and Olle Johansson. "Melanoma Incidence and Frequency Modulation (FM) Broadcasting." Archives of Environmental Health: An International Journal, vol. 57, no. 1, Jan. 2002, pp. 32–40. Crossref, doi: 10.1080/00039890209602914

23. Burch, J. B., et al. "Melatonin Metabolite Excretion among Cellular Telephone Users." International Journal of Radiation Biology, vol. 78, no. 11, Jan. 2002, pp. 1029–36. Crossref, doi: 10.1080/09553000210166561

24. Stevens, Richard G., and Scott Davis. "The Melatonin Hypothesis: Electric Power and Breast Cancer." Environmental Health Perspectives, vol. 104, Mar. 1996, p. 135. Crossref, doi: 10.2307/3432703

25. Wood, Brittany, et al. "Light Level and Duration of Exposure Determine the Impact of Self-Luminous Tablets on Melatonin Suppression." Applied Ergonomics, vol. 44, no. 2, Mar. 2013, pp. 237–40. Crossref, doi: 10.1016/j.apergo.2012.07.008

26. Pall, Martin L. "How to Approach the Challenge of Minimizing Non-Thermal Health Effects of Microwave Radiation from Electrical Devices." International Journal of Innovative Research in Engineering & Management (IJIREM), ISSN: 2350-557, vol. 2, no. 5, September 2015 https://www.researchgate.net/publication/283017154. (accessed 12 July 2018).

27. Pall, Martin L. "Electromagnetic Fields Act via Activation of Voltage-Gated Calcium Channels to Produce Beneficial or Adverse Effects." Journal of Cellular and Molecular Medicine, vol. 17, no. 8, Aug. 2013, pp. 958–65. Crossref, doi: 10.1111/jcmm.12088

28. Pall, Martin L. "Scientific Evidence Contradicts Findings and Assumptions of Canadian Safety Panel 6: Microwaves Act through Voltage-Gated Calcium Channel Activation to Induce Biological Impacts at Non-Thermal Levels, Supporting a Paradigm Shift for Microwave/Lower Frequency Electromagnetic Field Action." Reviews on Environmental Health, vol. 30, no. 2, Jan. 2015. Crossref, doi: 10.1515/reveh-2015-0001

29. Pall, Martin L. "Electromagnetic Fields Act Similarly in Plants as in Animals: Probable Activation of Calcium Channels via Their Voltage Sensor." Current Chemical Biology, vol. 10, no. 1, July 2016, pp. 74–82. Crossref, doi: 10.2174/2212796810666160419160433

30. Mortazavi, Ghazal, and S. M. J. Mortazavi. "Increased Mercury Release from Dental Amalgam Restorations after Exposure to Electromagnetic Fields as a Potential Hazard for Hypersensitive People and Pregnant Women." Reviews on Environmental Health, vol. 30, no. 4, Jan. 2015. Crossref, doi: 10.1515/reveh-2015-0017

31. Paknahad, Maryam, et al. "Effect of Radiofrequency Radiation from Wi-Fi Devices on Mercury Release from Amalgam Restorations." Journal of Environmental Health Science and Engineering, vol. 14, no. 1, Dec. 2016. Crossref, doi: 10.1186%2Fs40201-016-0253-z

32. Pall, Martin L. "Microwave Frequency Electromagnetic Fields (EMFs) Produce Widespread Neuropsychiatric Effects Including Depression." Journal of Chemical Neuroanatomy, vol. 75, Sept. 2016, pp. 43–51. Crossref, doi: 10.1016/j.jchemneu.2015.08.001

33. Milham, Samuel. "Historical Evidence that Electrification Caused the 20th Century Epidemic of 'Diseases of Civilization.'" Medical Hypotheses, vol. 74, no. 2, Feb. 2010, pp. 337–45. Crossref, doi: 10.1016/j.mehy.2009.08.032

34. Milham, Samuel. "Leukemia Clusters." Lancet (London, England), vol. 2, no. 7317, Nov. 1963, pp. 1122–23. Crossref, pmid: 14063438

35. Milham, S., and E. Ossiander. "Historical Evidence that Residential Electrification Caused the Emergence of the Childhood Leukemia Peak." Medical Hypotheses, vol. 56, no. 3, Mar. 2001, pp. 290–95. Crossref, doi: 10.1054/mehy.2000.1138

36. Milham, Samuel, and L. Lloyd Morgan. "A New Electromagnetic Exposure Metric: High Frequency Voltage Transients Associated with Increased Cancer Incidence in Teachers in a California School." American Journal of Industrial Medicine, vol. 51, no. 8, Aug. 2008, pp. 579–86. Crossref, doi: 10.1002/ajim.20598

37. Boardman Law Firm. "Wisconsin Supreme Court Upholds $1.2 Million Stray Voltage Judgment." Municipal Law Newsletter, Aug. 2003, www.boardmanclark.com/wordpress/wp-content/uploads/2012/01/muniAug03.pdf. (accessed 12 July 2018).

38. *Allan Hoffmann and Beverly Hoffmann vs. Wisconsin Electric Power Company*, 00-2703 WI 64 (2003) www.wicourts.gov/sc/opinions/pdf/00-2703.pdf. (accessed 12 July 2018).

39. "Stray Voltage." UW Milk Quality, https://milkquality.wisc.edu/milking-research-and-instruction/stray-voltage/. (accessed 12 July 2018).

40. Bawin, S. M., and W. R. Adey. "Sensitivity of Calcium Binding in Cerebral Tissue to Weak Environmental Electric Fields Oscillating at Low Frequency." Proceedings of the National Academy of Sciences of the United States of America, vol. 73, no. 6, June 1976, pp. 1999–2003. Crossref, pmid: 1064869

41. Hendee, S. P., et al. "The Effects of Weak Extremely Low Frequency Magnetic Fields on Calcium/Calmodulin Interactions." Biophysical Journal, vol. 70, no. 6, June 1996, pp. 2915–23. Crossref, doi: 10.1016/S0006-3495(96)79861-2

42. Lerchl, Alexander, et al. "Evidence That Extremely Low Frequency Ca2+-Cyclotron Resonance Depresses Pineal Melatonin Synthesis in Vitro." Neuroscience Letters, vol. 124, no. 2, Apr. 1991, pp. 213–15. Crossref, doi: 10.1016/0304-3940(91)90096-C

43. Grellier, James, et al. "Potential Health Impacts of Residential Exposures to Extremely Low Frequency Magnetic Fields in Europe." Environment International, vol. 62, Jan. 2014, pp. 55–63. Crossref, doi: 10.1016/j.envint.2013.09.017

44. Soffritti, Morando, et al. "Life-Span Exposure to Sinusoidal-50 Hz Magnetic Field and Acute Low-Dose γ Radiation Induce Carcinogenic Effects in Sprague-Dawley Rats." International Journal of Radiation Biology, vol. 92, no. 4, Apr. 2016, pp. 202–14. Crossref, doi: 10.3109/09553002.2016.1144942

45. Stevens, Richard G., and Scott Davis. "The Melatonin Hypothesis: Electric Power and Breast Cancer." Environmental Health Perspectives, vol. 104, 1996, pp. 135–40. JSTOR. Crossref, doi: 0.2307/3432703

46. Wilson, Bary W., et al. "Chronic Exposure to 60-Hz Electric Fields: Effects on Pineal Function in the Rat." Bioelectromagnetics, vol. 2, no. 4, 1981, pp. 371–80. Crossref, doi: 10.1002/bem.2250020408

47. Lee, Jong Hun, et al. "Dietary Phytochemicals and Cancer Prevention: Nrf2 Signaling, Epigenetics, and Cell Death Mechanisms in Blocking Cancer Initiation and Progression." Pharmacology & Therapeutics, vol. 137, no. 2, Feb. 2013, pp. 153–71. Crossref, doi: 10.1016/j.pharmthera.2012.09.008

48. Blask, David, et al. "Melatonin as a Chronobiotic / Anticancer Agent: Cellular, Biochemical, and Molecular Mechanisms of Action and Their Implications for Circadian-Based Cancer Therapy." Current Topics in Medicinal Chemistry, vol. 2, no. 2, Feb. 2002, pp. 113–32. Crossref, doi: 10.2174/1568026023394407

49. Dorfman, Ariel. "The Whispering Leaves of the Hiroshima Ginkgo Trees." The New York Times, 4 Aug. 2017. NYTimes.com, https://www.nytimes.com/2017/08/04/opinion/the-whispering-leaves-of-the-hiroshima-ginkgo-trees.html. (accessed 12 July 2018).

50. Ilhan, Atilla, et al. "Ginkgo Biloba Prevents Mobile Phone-Induced Oxidative Stress in Rat Brain." Clinica Chimica Acta, vol. 340, no. 1–2, Feb. 2004, pp. 153–62. Crossref, doi: 10.1016/j.cccn.2003.10.012

51. Gray, Janet M., et al. "State of the Evidence 2017: An Update on the Connection between Breast Cancer and the Environment." Environmental Health, vol. 16, no. 1, Dec. 2017. Crossref, doi: 10.1186/s12940-017-0287-4

52. iPad, Environmental Health Trust. "How to Connect Your Device to the Ethernet." It Takes Time, 9 June 2015, http://it-takes-time.com/2015/06/09/how-to-connect-device-to-the-ethernet/. (accessed 12 July 2018).

53. Lamech, Federica. "Self-Reporting of Symptom Development from Exposure to Radiofrequency Fields of Wireless Smart Meters in Victoria, Australia: A Case Series." Alternative Therapies in Health and Medicine, vol. 20, no. 6, Dec. 2014, pp. 28–39. Crossref, pmid: 25478801

54. Maine Department of Environmental Protection. "Maine Compact Fluorescent Lamp Breakage Study Report." Feb. 2008, http://www11.maine.gov/dep/homeowner/cflreport.html. (accessed 12 July 2018).

55. Sinatra, Stephen T., et al. "Electric Nutrition: The Surprising Health and Healing Benefits of Biological Grounding (Earthing)." Alternative Therapies in Health and Medicine, vol. 23, no. 5, Sept. 2017, pp. 8–16. Crossref, pmid: 28987038

56. Passi R, Doheny K, K, Gordin Y, Hinssen H, Palmer C, "Electrical Grounding Improves Vagal Tone in Preterm Infants." Neonatology 2017;112:187–192. Crossref, doi: 10.1159/000475744

57. National Toxicology Program. "Definition of Carcinogenicity Results." https://ntp.niehs.nih.gov/go/baresults. (accessed 12 July 2018).

58. National Toxicology Program. Abstract for TR-596. "Toxicology and Carcinogenesis Studies in B6C3F1/N Mice Exposed to Whole-Body Radio Frequency Radiation at a Frequency (1,900 MHz) and Modulations (GSM and CDMA) Used by Cell Phones." https://www.niehs.nih.gov/ntp-temp/ tr596_508.pdf. (accessed 5 November 2018).

59. National Toxicology Program. Abstract for TR-595. "Toxicology and Carcinogenesis Studies in Hsd:Sprague Dawley SD Rats Exposed to Whole-Body Radio Frequency Radiation at a Frequency (900 MHz) and Modulations (GSM and CDMA) Used by Cell Phones." https://www.niehs.nih.gov/ ntp-temp/tr595_508.pdf. (accessed 5 November 2018).

60. National Toxicology Program. "Actions from Peer Review of the Draft NTP Technical Reports on Cell Phone Radiofrequency Radiation March 26-28, 2018." https://ntp.niehs.nih. gov/ntp/about_ntp/trpanel/2018/march/ actions20180328_508.pdf. (accessed 5 November 2018).

61. BioInitiative Report. "BioInitiative 2012: A Rationale for a Biologically-Based Public Exposure Standard for Electromagnetic Fields (ELF and RF)." http://www.bioinitiative.org/. (accessed 12 July 2018).

62. American Cancer Society. "Lifetime Risk of Developing or Dying From Cancer." https://www.cancer.org/cancer/cancer-basics/lifetime-probability-of-developing-or-dying-from-cancer.html. (accessed 12 July 2018).

63. Cancer Research UK. "Why Are Cancer Rates Increasing?" Science Blog, http://scienceblog.cancerresearchuk.org/2015/02/04/why-are-cancer-rates-increasing/. (accessed 12 July 2018).

64. Chowdhury, Rajiv, et al. "Association of Dietary, Circulating, and Supplement Fatty Acids With Coronary Risk: A Systematic Review and Meta-Analysis." Annals of Internal Medicine, vol. 160, no. 6, Mar. 2014, p. 398. Crossref, doi: 10.7326/M13-1788

65. De-Sola Gutiérrez, José, Fernando Rodríguez de Fonseca, and Gabriel Rubio. "Cell-Phone Addiction: A Review." Frontiers in Psychiatry 7 (2016). Crossref, doi: 10.3389/fpsyt.2016.00175